RAND NATIONAL DEFENSE RESEARCH INSTITUTE

Personnel Recovery in the AFRICOM Area of Responsibility

Cost-Effective Options for Improvement

Christopher A. Mouton, Edward W. Chan, Adam R. Grissom,
John P. Godges, Badreddine Ahtchi, Brian Dougherty

Prepared for the U.S. Africa Command (AFRICOM)

Approved for public release; distribution unlimited

For more information on this publication, visit www.rand.org/t/RR2161z1

Library of Congress Cataloging-in-Publication Data is available for this publication.
ISBN: 978-1-9774-0145-8

Published by the RAND Corporation, Santa Monica, Calif.
© Copyright 2019 RAND Corporation
RAND® is a registered trademark.

Support RAND
Make a tax-deductible charitable contribution at
www.rand.org/giving/contribute

www.rand.org

Preface

This report updates ongoing research on the mission of rescuing injured personnel in Africa. Previous work called for a new approach to this mission, and this report offers such an approach. The objective is to identify the most cost-effective options for improving rescue capabilities in the U.S. Africa Command (AFRICOM) area of responsibility.

This research was sponsored by David Thiede of AFRICOM and conducted within the Acquisition and Technology Policy Center of the RAND National Defense Research Institute, a federally funded research and development center sponsored by the Office of the Secretary of Defense, the Joint Staff, the Unified Combatant Commands, the Navy, the Marine Corps, the defense agencies, and the defense Intelligence Community.

For more information on the Acquisition and Technology Policy Center, see www.rand.org/nsrd/ndri/centers/atp, or contact the director (contact information is provided on the webpage).

Contents

Figures and Tables

Figures

Tables

DATAMATION IMAGING SERVICES

BOOKS RECEIVING

SHIP
TO: 7700 GRIFFIN WAY STE B

WILLOWBROOK

IL   60527

US

ORDER NO.	DATE	PAGE NO.
1123-082312312	09/09/24	1 of 1

SHIPMENT NO.	SHIP VIA
ETZ0949097U	Varies

Item Number	SHIP	Line	Item Description	Ord	Purchase Order No.
9781958211441	1	000005	Patient	1	1123-082312312
9781977404039	1	000072	Navigating Current and Emerging Army Recruiting Challenges	1	1123-082312312
9781977405241	1	000082	Frameworks for Assessing Useucom Efforts to Inform, Influence, and Persuade	1	1123-082312312
9781987915082	1	000200	The Dirty Knees of Prayer	1	1123-082312312
9781977405555	1	000086	Options for Ensuring Safe Elections	1	1123-082312312
9781977412256	1	000125	U.S.-Japan Alliance Conference	1	1123-082312312
9781977403452	1	000064	Understanding Russian Black Sea Power Dynamics Through National Security Gaming	1	1123-082312312
9781977406095	1	000089	Developing Operationally Relevant Metrics for Measuring and Tracking Readiness in the U.S.	1	1123-082312312
9781977402493	1	000056	The Project May Serve the Nation - But What About Us, Who Live Here?	1	1123-082312312
9781977401953	1	000045	Trends in Russia's Armed Forces	1	1123-082312312
9781977404343	1	000075	A New Zimbabwe?	1	1123-082312312
9781977405364	1	000084	Command and Control in U.S. Naval Competition with China	1	1123-082312312
9781977406453	1	000090	Can Artificial Intelligence Help Improve Air Force Talent Management?	1	1123-082312312
9781977407528	1	000105	Commercial and Military Applications and Timelines for Quantum Technology	1	1123-082312312
9781987915228	1	000202	Acquired Community	1	1123-082312312
9781977401458	1	000037	Personnel Recovery in the AFRICOM Area of Responsibility	1	1123-082312312
9781977401588	1	000041	Overcoming Challenges Arising from the Creation of National Security Councils	1	1123-082312312
9781977401830	1	000043	Alternative Paths to Korean Unification	1	1123-082312312
9781977406828	1	000097	Talent Management for U.S. Department of Defense Knowledge Workers	1	1123-082312312
9781977407498	1	000104	AI Tools for Military Readiness	1	1123-082312312
9781987915204	1	000201	The Day of the Dead	1	1123-082312312
9781977400598	1	000028	Charting Progress	1	1123-082312312
9781977408358	1	000012	Forecasting Public Recovery Expenditures' Effect on Construction Prices and the Demand for	1	1123-082312312
9781977412881	1	000127	Attributing Biological Weapons Use	1	1123-082312312
9781977404015	1	000070	Gaming Gray Zone Tactics	1	1123-082312312

Return Label

VIA:

SHIPPER NO.

PKG. ID# **100117787**

ORDER # 1123-082312123

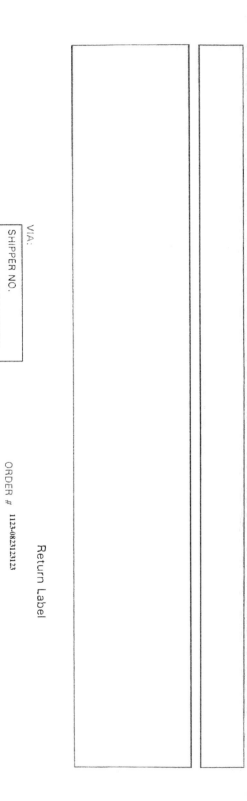

Summary

This report updates ongoing research on the mission of rescuing injured personnel in Africa. Previous work called for a new approach to this mission, and this report offers such an approach. The objective is to identify the most cost-effective options for improving rescue capabilities in the U.S. Africa Command (AFRICOM) area of responsibility (AOR).

The Rescue Model

To compare the cost-effectiveness of additional rescue investments, we built a model that accounts for the following seven factors:

- the costs of new rescue capabilities
- the current and projected locations of medical treatment facilities (MTFs) in AFRICOM
- the current and projected locations of deployed aircraft in Africa
- the existing locations of airfields in Africa
- the locations and numbers of U.S. personnel in Africa
- the survival rates of injured personnel as a function of time and of medical care received
- the trends in injury occurrences in combat theaters.

The model allows us to estimate, for a given population deployed in Africa, the marginal cost-effectiveness of alternative investments that are designed to raise the survivability rates for injured personnel. Figure S.1 diagrams the model, showing the capability costs on the left, the "rescue capability" inputs across the top, and the "personnel injury" inputs across the bottom.

Figure S.1
Diagram of Rescue Model Inputs

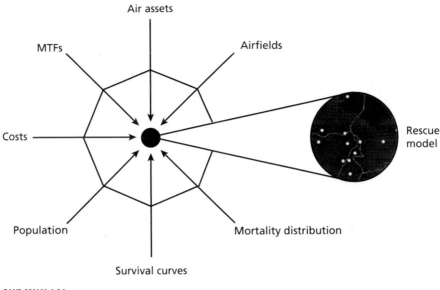

Cost Analysis

One implication of the unique operating environment of Africa is that the capabilities best suited to fulfilling AFRICOM's rescue requirements are themselves unique in terms of their organizational and budgetary requirements. Because of this uniqueness, we were unable to find reliable cost data and instead investigated analogous commercial services for estimating the costs of the unique military capabilities.

We use commercial cost analogies for four alternative components of a rescue capability: a pair (or "node") of light fixed-wing aircraft, a pair of medium rotary-wing aircraft, a fixed damage control surgery (DCS) team (a patient is moved to the DCS location), or a mobile DCS team (a DCS team can move to the patient location).[1] Given the uncertainty of the individual cost estimates and the diversity of the underlying data, the estimates are best understood as scoping benchmarks rather than point predictions of actual costs. We recommend that AFRICOM use a round scoping factor of $10 million as an annual cost estimate for each of the four alternative components of a rescue capability: the fixed-wing airlift node, the rotary-wing airlift node, the fixed DCS team, and the mobile DCS team. In all four cases, the annual marginal

---

[1]   We use the term *DCS* to emphasize that these teams are smaller and more mobile—focused on damage control surgery as opposed to surgery more broadly—than the forward surgical teams (FSTs) or expeditionary medical support teams deployed during Operation Enduring Freedom and Operation Iraqi Freedom.

cost would be roughly $10 million, with potential costs ranging from $5 million to $20 million per year.

Given the uncertainty in the actual cost distribution, we note the approximate equivalence of the estimated cost of each of the four alternative additional elements of a rescue capability. Although each one would play a distinct role in enhancing AFRICOM's rescue capabilities, the cost of each component could be comparable within a very broad range of uncertainty. Because of the approximate similarity of costs across the four investment options, we simplify the cost-effectiveness analysis to come, reducing it to an analysis of effectiveness.

"Rescue Capability" Inputs

The three "effectiveness" variables across the top of the model diagram consist of "rescue capability" inputs. These represent the rescue resources that currently exist in Africa or could be added there. The inputs include MTFs, air assets, and airfields.

Broadly speaking, medical professionals in AFRICOM perform two categories of medical care that are pertinent to rescue missions in Africa: first responder care and DCS.[2] In general, first responder care is the only care initially available for injured personnel in the field, whereas DCS is available once injured personnel are moved to an MTF or a DCS team is moved to the persons locations.

The baseline AFRICOM rescue capability inputs for our model include MTF locations, basing locations with air assets, and hundreds of airfields of varying maximum demonstrated capabilities. In addition, 32 host-nation hospitals in 20 African cities could potentially be utilized for trauma care when it could not otherwise be provided by U.S. or allied MTFs. Because of the danger of the blood supply at host-nation hospitals throughout the continent, we assess them as unacceptable for force planning purposes and recommend that they should be utilized *in extremis*, when no better option is available.

"Personnel Injury" Inputs

The three "effectiveness" variables across the bottom of the model diagram consist of 'personnel injury' inputs. These include population at risk (PAR), survival curves, and mortality risk distributions. These inputs feed into our construction of average survival timelines, which establish the expected survival rates over time for personnel receiving different levels of care for different severities of life-threatening injuries.

---

[2] First responder care and DCS encompass five of the seven roles of care in the U.S. military's Joint Medical Planning Tool (JMPT) (Teledyne Brown Engineering, Inc., 2015). We consolidate some roles to distinguish more clearly between the levels of care associated with rescue missions.

Figure S.2 shows the PAR. The geographic dispersion of the PAR greatly affects the survival benefits, as estimated in the model, of adding aviation or medical assets in different locations.

Figure S.2
Geographic Dispersion of Population at Risk

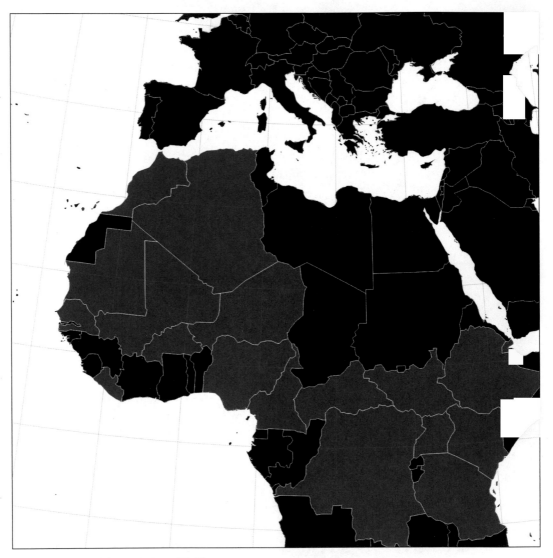

SOURCE: Adapted from McCann (2018).
RAND *RR2161z1-S.2*

The second personnel injury input is a set of survival curves that vary according to the severity of injury suffered, the level of care administered, and the amount of time spent at each level of care. These survival curves are drawn from the Joint Medical Planning Tool (JMPT) (Teledyne Brown Engineering, Inc., 2015). The JMPT assigns to hundreds of patients' conditions the probability distribution of causing four different levels of mortality risk. Three of the risk levels indicate that a condition is life-threatening (with either a high, medium, or low mortality risk), while the fourth risk level indicates that the condition is non-life-threatening. Because each condition code can be assigned to no more than four mortality risk levels, it is the distribution among the four risks—and not the distribution among the hundreds of injuries or conditions—that we use in our mortality modeling.

The third personnel injury input is the historical distribution of injuries suffered at each mortality risk level. The mortality risk distribution data are drawn from the Medical Planners' Toolkit (MPTk) (Naval Health Research Center, 2013). We focus on 15 historical MPTk datasets representing a range of locations and conflict conditions over the past 50 years. As it turns out, the results prove to be insensitive to the precise nature of each conflict. There is a surprising consistency across the historical events: For any person who has received a life-threatening injury in conflict, there has consistently been about a 25-percent chance that the injury will pose a high mortality risk, a 25-percent chance that it will pose a medium mortality risk, and a 50-percent chance that it will pose a low mortality risk.

Using the historical distribution of mortality risks, we can ascertain the weighted average survival rates across the conflict scenarios. The weighted average survival rates depend, of course, on the levels of care received by personnel facing the different mortality risks. The weighted average survival rates for two different levels of care can be seen in the two survival curves in Figure S.3.[3] The lower curve is for first responder care; the higher curve is for DCS. Each curve shows the weighted average expected survival rate, from hour to hour, for any patient with a life-threatening injury of any severity level receiving the specified care level in any of the historical conflict scenarios considered or in any future conflict scenario. Thus, by combining the geographic distribution of the PAR with the survival curves from the JMPT and the historical mortality risk data from the MPTk, we can predict the average percentage of injured personnel who will likely survive under varying "rescue capability" conditions and time frames.

---

[3]   These survival curves provide the analytic basis for quantifying the benefits of improved rescue times in terms of patient outcomes.

Figure S.3
Weighted Average Survival Curves

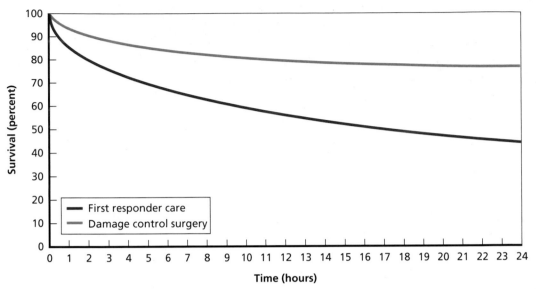

SOURCE: Teledyne Brown Engineering Inc., 2015.
RAND RR2161z1-S.3

Rescue Model Outputs

The rescue model generates two types of outputs: optimal rescue paths and optimal asset-location pairings. The optimal rescue paths are the most life-saving routes to various levels of medical care from anywhere on the continent. The optimal asset-location pairings are the most cost-effective marginal investments in rescue capabilities. In the model, each additional investment option is paired with an airfield location, yielding a succession of optimal asset-location pairings, in order of diminishing marginal cost-effectiveness.

The model charts alternative rescue paths as a first step toward estimating the survival rates that could be expected from different response speeds and care levels. Figure S.4 shows a purely notional example of a rescue path for an individual injured in the Central African Republic. For each path, the model also computes the average statistics for incident response times, travel times to a DCS team, and survival rates, depending on the mortality risks incurred and the care level (or role of care) administered.

To identify the optimal asset-location pairings, the model calculates the marginal effectiveness (in terms of raising the expected survival rates) of investing in four separate rescue assets at separate African basing locations while instituting two separate aircraft alert times. Once the first optimal additional asset is placed at its respective location, the model seeks the next optimal additional asset-location pairing, and so on.

Figure S.4
Optimal Rescue Path and Expected Survival (Notional)

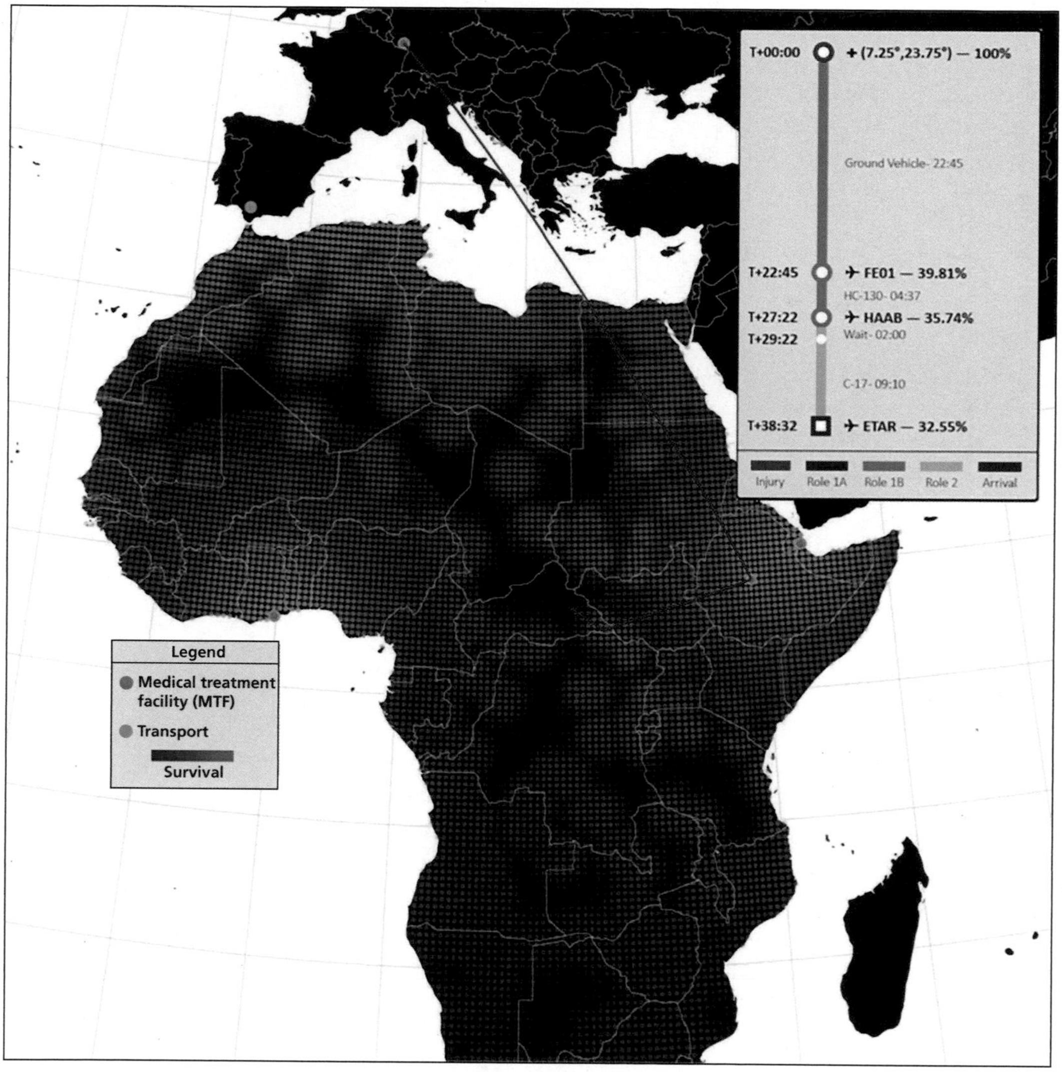

NOTE: Survival rates, MTFs, and transports displayed in the figure are notional and for illustrative purposes only.

RAND RR2161z1-S.4

Figure S.5 summarizes the results from thousands of model runs premised on varying sets of assumptions. (In the case of zero additional assets, these curves show the benefit of decreasing the alert times of existing aircraft and/or making current DCS capabilities mobile.)

The results in Figure S.5 all appear within the "survival window" of "baseline risk" and "minimum risk," which represent the most full range of rescue capabilities available to AFRICOM today. The four alternative rescue assets are, as mentioned

Figure S.5
Optimal Additional Assets, Under Different Sets of Assumptions

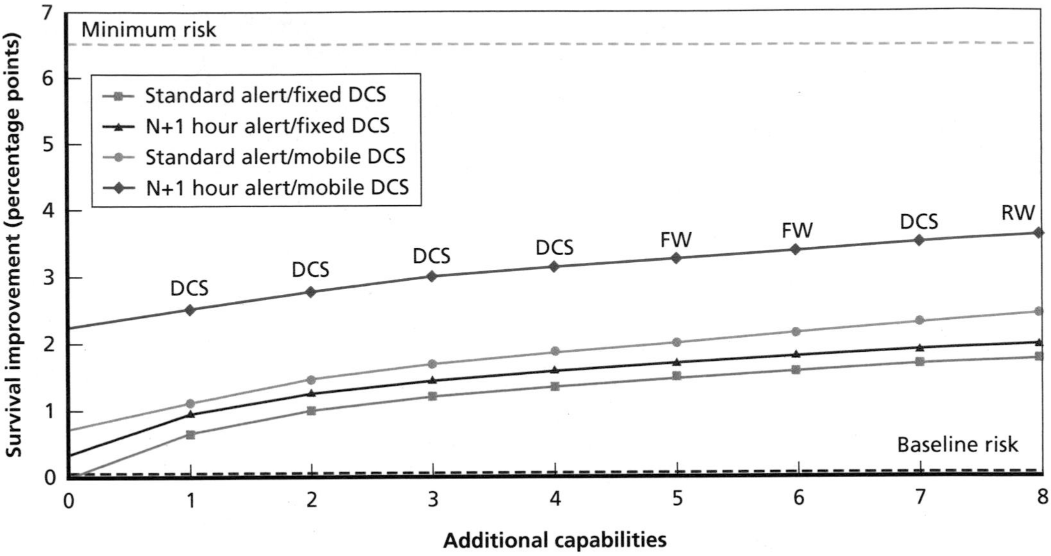

NOTES: DCS = damage control surgery; FW = fixed-wing; RW = rotary-wing.
RAND RR2161z1-S.5

above, a light fixed-wing aircraft node, a medium rotary-wing aircraft node, a fixed DCS team, and a mobile DCS team. The two aircraft alert times are the assumed standard N+3 (three-hour notice) and the accelerated N+1 (one-hour notice). The figure shows a relatively large jump in expected survival rates from combining the shorter alert times with the mobile DCS capability. In fact, even without a single additional asset, mobile DCS teams combined with shortened alert times produces an equal or better outcome than all eight optimal additional investments under the other sets of conditions.

Three key findings emerge from our comparisons of the cost-effectiveness of rescue investment options:

1. There is a very strong synergy to be gained from combining mobile DCS teams with shorter aircraft alert times (e.g., N+1).
2. These synergies increase rapidly with decreasing alert times below one hour. Compared with a notional alert time of three hours, an alert time of 15 minutes would be more than twice as beneficial as an alert time of one hour. The expected survival rate would rise 1.5 percentage points going from three hours' notice to one hour's notice and 3.4 percentage points going from three hours' notice to 15 minutes' notice.
3. Under all sets of conditions considered, additional DCS teams are always initially preferred to additional aircraft.

Recommendations

This analysis points toward three recommendations for AFRICOM regarding cost-effective options for improving rescue, as follows:

1. Coordinate with DCS providers (Air Combat Command, Air Force Special Operations Command, Air Mobility Command, Army Medical Department, Navy Bureau of Medicine, and others) to ensure that mobile DCS teams can move surgical capabilities to patients during rescue missions.
2. Decrease the alert times of dedicated rescue aircraft to one hour.
3. Explore the feasibility of decreasing the alert times to less than one hour. The times can vary by location and can be adjusted, based on the estimated risk to force. The rescue aircraft and DCS teams can also be forward-staged to support high-risk activities in high-intensity zones of operation. These are just some of the options that can be explored.

Acknowledgments

We are extremely appreciative of the ongoing support we receive from AFRICOM. In particular, we would like to thank the project sponsor, David Thiede, as well as LTC Marv King, CDR Michael Kamas, and Maj David Risius. Their insights, suggestions, and willingness to help were pivotal in the performance of this work. We also thank CDR Byron Wiggins, Robert Shellenberger, and Lt Col Donovan Cirino for their continuing support.

We would like to thank both Brig Gen Lee Payne and Col Linda Guerrero for their insights and feedback throughout this research. Col Mark Ervin provided invaluable information on medical capabilities and challenges. We are also very appreciative of the big picture insight that both Maj Gen Joseph Caravalho and COL Christopher Lettieri provided. The feedback that we received from Maj Gen Roosevelt Allen and his team helped us further refine our research.

At RAND, we thank Sherban Drulea and Russell Hanson for their amazing and invaluable work, and Damien Baveye for helping put together this abridged version. We would like to acknowledge the excellent management support we received from Cynthia Cook. Finally, we would like to thank Brent Thomas for his highly constructive reviews of this work, as well as Brad DeBlois and Steve Dalzell for their reviews of previous work that served as a foundation for this effort.

Abbreviations

AE	aeromedical evacuation
AFRICOM	U.S. Africa Command
AOR	area of responsibility
CASEVAC	casualty evacuation
COA	course of action
DCS	damage control surgery
DHA	Defense Health Agency
DoD	U.S. Department of Defense
EAP	emergency action plan
FST	forward surgical team
FW	fixed-wing
GARS	Global Area Reference System
HCV	hepatitis C virus
HIV	human immunodeficiency virus
HNV	hematopoietic necrosis virus
ICD-9	*International Classification of Diseases, 9th Revision*
JCI	Joint Commission International
JMPT	Joint Medical Planning Tool
JP	Joint Publication
MEDEVAC	medical evacuation
MFST	mobile field surgical team
MPTk	Medical Planners' Toolkit
MTF	medical treatment facility
NCMI	National Center for Medical Intelligence
OEF	Operation Enduring Freedom
OIF	Operation Iraqi Freedom

PAR	population at risk
PR	personnel recovery
RFI	request for information
role 2E	role 2 enhanced
RW	rotary-wing
SOST	Special Operations Surgical Team
TCCET-E	Tactical Critical Care Evacuation Team-Enhanced
TOP	TRICARE Overseas Program
TSSA	Trauma Society of South Africa
WHO	World Health Organization

CHAPTER ONE

Introduction

This report continues a stream of ongoing research on the mission of rescuing injured personnel in Africa, an important and demanding component of personnel recovery (PR) operations in the theater. Previous work called for a new approach to accomplishing this mission, and this report offers such an approach. This chapter describes the motivation for the ongoing research, connects the previous work to the latest work, summarizes the analytical approach presented here, offers some caveats, and outlines the remainder of this report.

Motivation

The operational challenges confronting U.S. Africa Command (AFRICOM) make PR, medical evacuation (MEDEVAC), casualty evacuation (CASEVAC), and aero-medical evacuation (AE)—which we collectively term *rescue* for purposes of this analysis—uniquely difficult but increasingly important.[1] The limited scale yet widely

---

[1] There is disagreement within the U.S. Department of Defense (DoD) over the appropriate doctrinal terminology to apply to the mission of rescuing personnel who are injured or wounded away from U.S. facilities in Africa. AFRICOM refers to this mission as *personnel recovery*. This is a plausible interpretation because of the semipermissive conditions in the active operational areas of the continent, areas in which any personnel injured away from base would seem to meet the definition of isolated personnel in Department of Defense Directive 3002.01, *Personnel Recovery in the Department of Defense* (2017):

> U.S. military, DoD civilians and contractor personnel (and others designated by the President or Secretary of Defense) who are separated from their unit (as an individual or a group) while participating in a U.S. sponsored military activity or mission and are, or may be, in a situation *where they must survive, evade, resist, or escape.* (emphasis added)

On the other hand, Joint Publication (JP) 3-50, *Personnel Recovery* (2017), clearly excludes both MEDEVAC and CASEVAC from PR, and some on the Joint Staff likewise insist that AFRICOM's requirements do not meet the formal "wartime" definition of PR (JP 3-50). Our assessment is that AFRICOM's operational conditions are incongruent with the bright lines drawn between war and peace in JP 3-50. On balance, we assess that personnel injured away from U.S. facilities in Africa meet the definition of isolated personnel and that their rescue is best understood as a form of PR. To reflect the ambiguity of the doctrinal fit, however, we have coined the term *medical rescue* to encompass all aspects of the mission, whether they be categorized as PR, MEDEVAC, CASEVAC, AE, or another doctrinal term.

distributed nature of AFRICOM's operations, its semipermissive security conditions across key operational areas, and the ambiguities of kinetic activity outside declared theaters of active armed conflict (ODTAAC) all combine to create rescue requirements in AFRICOM that do not conform neatly to joint doctrine or the assumptions implicit in DoD's processes for joint operational planning, capability development, and global force management.[2] Meanwhile, the growing ambition of U.S. national objectives for countering terrorism on the continent, and the resulting risks to mission and force, make the ability to rescue injured personnel particularly important. Together, the difficulty and importance create a situation in which the rescue requirements are rapidly becoming more demanding yet one in which a failure to recover an injured person could jeopardize the strategic approach in the region. Effective rescue capabilities are therefore of strategic importance to AFRICOM and DoD. Without effective rescue capabilities, the U.S. strategic presence in Africa might not be possible at all.

Therefore, in 2016, AFRICOM asked RAND to conduct an analysis of rescue requirements and options. The objective of this analysis is to identify the most cost-effective options for improving rescue capabilities in the AFRICOM area of responsibility (AOR). This analysis assumes that the scale and nature of future deployment patterns, future threat patterns, and future rescue events across Africa will be similar to those of recent standard practices and experiences in Africa and elsewhere. This report codifies the results of the analysis.

To compare the cost-effectiveness of additional rescue investments, we built a model that simulates the effects of prevailing conditions, including the costs of new rescue capabilities, the locations and numbers of U.S. personnel in Africa, the trends in injury occurrences in combat theaters, the survival rates of injured personnel as a function of time and of medical care received, and the current and projected locations of rescue assets, from medical treatment facilities (MTFs) to deployed aircraft to existing airfields. This model allows us to estimate, for a given population deployed on the continent, how much additional rescue capabilities could raise the overall survivability rates. We then compare the alternative investments in rescue capabilities on the basis of their marginal cost-effectiveness.

Previous Research

In our previous research on rescue missions in Africa (not available to the general public), we developed survivability timelines as a basis for assessing rescue options

---

2   *Semipermissive security conditions* refers to the uncertain environment that exists throughout much of the AFRICOM AOR, where *uncertain environment* is defined by an "operational environment in which host government forces, whether opposed to or receptive to operations that a unit intends to conduct, do not have totally effective control of the territory and population in the intended operational area" (U.S. Department of Defense, 2016).

either for Africa as a whole or for specific regions (Mouton, Godges, and Chan, 2018). These timelines accounted for several inputs: the distribution of the population at risk (PAR), the distribution of rescue capabilities, the historical distribution of life-threatening injuries, and the mortality risks associated with those injuries. These inputs determined the baseline, or expected, survival rates for injured personnel over time. The survivability timelines highlighted how quickly the expected survival rates fell over the course of just a few hours.

The findings also underscored the unique challenges posed by the African context—the vast distances, the dispersed personnel, and the limited rescue capabilities—thus requiring a unique solution as well. These results were fairly consistent across a wide range of assumptions. In particular, the expected survival rates—across historical, operational, and clinical cases—were relatively insensitive to the rescue times whenever the rescue times exceeded four to six hours.

Figure 1.1 shows why Africa is different and why it requires a different approach. DoD's traditional approach to rescuing personnel is typified by the robust rescue postures in Iraq and Afghanistan. This traditional approach is premised on the realities of large numbers of personnel facing life-threatening injuries, and on those injuries occurring at high rates across relatively small geographic areas, resulting in highly dense pockets of major trauma injuries. But Africa represents the opposite extremes in almost all of these respects. In Africa, small numbers of personnel face life-threatening injuries, and those injuries thankfully occur at much lower rates but across an enormous geographic expanse, resulting in low-density, widely dispersed injuries.

The ramifications of the thought exercise in Figure 1.1 are stark. Even if AFRICOM today were provided all of the rescue assets that were deployed to Afghanistan during the U.S. surge in Operation Enduring Freedom (OEF), the average time across the AOR for rescuing injured personnel in Africa and delivering them to surgical facilities would still be seven hours—well beyond the survivability window for many injured

Figure 1.1
Across the Board, Africa Is the Opposite of Iraq and Afghanistan

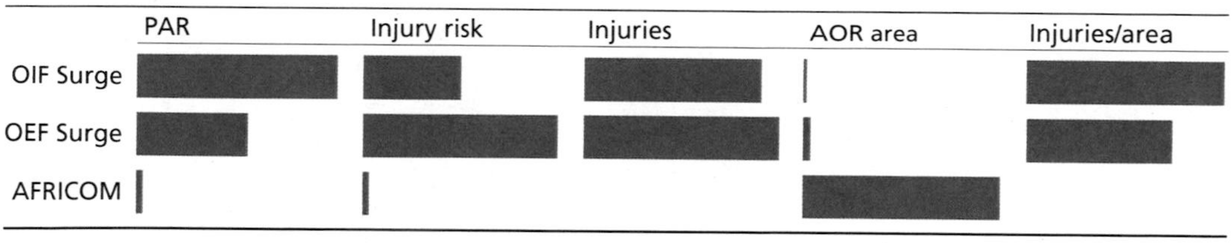

NOTES: OIF = Operation Iraqi Freedom; OEF = Operating Enduring Freedom. Each bar is to scale, with the maximum case representing a full bar. The total number of AFRICOM injuries is too small to be visible when scaled to the OEF Surge injury number.
RAND RR2161z1-1.1

personnel, including some with relatively minor life-threatening injuries.[3] Moreover, even with all of the assets simultaneously deployed to support operations in Iraq and Afghanistan, AFRICOM would still not be able to achieve rapid rescue times. Thus, in the rescue domain, as in many others, operational effectiveness in AFRICOM requires a different approach than what has been pursued in other theaters.

The earlier RAND research (Mouton, Godges, and Chan, 2018) compared a limited set of potential courses of action (COAs) for improving survival rates in rescue missions. These COAs were meant to span the range of possible solutions: adding a paramedic to existing aircraft, investing in additional rescue aircraft, deploying a mobile surgical capability (so that surgical care could be flown to a patient), and decreasing the alert times of rescue aircraft. The most effective of these COAs was to deploy a mobile surgical capability on the continent. The second most effective COA, of those examined, was to decrease the alert time of rescue aircraft. In contrast, the least effective COAs were to invest in additional rescue aircraft or to add a paramedic to existing rescue aircraft.

The previous results are consistent with our current analysis. In particular, the greatest expected improvements in survival rates come from *combining* mobile surgical capabilities with decreased alert times. This research reported here focuses on identifying the most cost-effective combinations of these two improvements.

Analytical Approach

Figure 1.2 offers an overview of our methodology, showing the seven inputs that feed into our rescue model. The "costs" on the far left of the figure represent the estimated marginal costs of four alternative rescue asset options that we consider in this analysis: light fixed-wing aircraft, medium rotary-wing aircraft, fixed damage control surgery (DCS) teams, and mobile DCS teams. The other six factors in the rescue model are the "effectiveness" inputs. Across the top of the figure are three "rescue capability" inputs: MTFs, air assets (aircraft), and airfields. Across the bottom of the figure are three "personnel injury" inputs: PAR, survival curves, and mortality risk distributions. Together, the rescue capabilities and the personnel risks generate the outputs of the model in terms of effectiveness, specifically the rescue times and survival rates. When the effectiveness outputs are divided by the cost inputs, the model indicates the cost-effectiveness of each additional capability.

---

[3]   See Mouton, Godges, and Chan (2018) for additional discussion on this comparison.

Figure 1.2
Inputs to the Rescue Model of Cost-Effectiveness

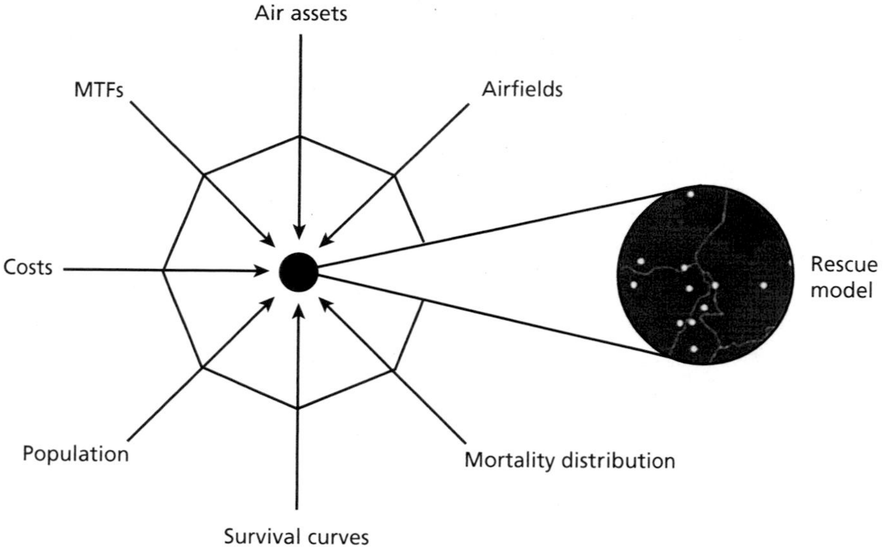

Air assets

MTFs

Airfields

Costs

Rescue model

Population

Mortality distribution

Survival curves

Caveats

Our analysis indicates that our findings are robust against a wide set of assumptions. Nevertheless, it is important to discuss the limitations of the analysis and to offer four caveats.

First, this work is focused primarily on what we call *rescue*, which we define as currently the most pressing subset of PR in the AFRICOM AOR. However, PR includes rescues beyond those of a medical nature. By definition, PR encompasses personnel rescues of all types that must be conducted in nonpermissive and unstable environments. The spectrum of such events, from rescuing a downed pilot to retrieving civilians from a besieged hotel, requires a spectrum of specialized capabilities, many of which are not captured in this analysis.

Second, there may be personnel at locations in Africa who are not fully reflected or accurately captured in the personnel statistics on which our analysis is based. Initial indications suggest that the number of personnel in this category is very small, and so it is unlikely to affect the broad geographic pattern of personnel. At the same time, these undisclosed personnel might not be co-located with airfields, which could change the rescue dynamics and perhaps require more rotary-wing lift than indicated by our rescue model.

Third, this analysis treats all personnel as being at equal risk. We made this assumption primarily because of a lack of available data and thus the need to rely on "average" levels of risk. However, we know from historical data that operating locations and the operational activities of personnel can have very large effects on the differential levels of individual personnel risk. For example, the risk to U.S. personnel in Iraq over the past decade varied by an order of magnitude based solely on the branch of service to which the personnel belonged (Preston and Buzzell, 2006). In a similar vein, it is easy to imagine that a soldier engaged in a counterterrorism operation could face a much higher level of individual risk than would an airman working the flight line at Djibouti airfield.

Fourth and finally, the scope of potential improvements to AFRICOM's rescue posture is limited in this analysis to solutions that seemed most promising at the time of this research. Therefore, this analysis does not consider broader improvements to medical care that could fundamentally shift the survival curves upward. These improvements could include, but are certainly not limited to, enhancing the initial medical care delivered; providing a theater hospital (role 3 care) somewhere on the African continent; or providing more responsive, but nonsurgical, resuscitative care.

Organization of This Report

As illustrated in Figure 1.2, the rescue model compares the costs of additional rescue capabilities with their effectiveness, as predicted by three rescue capability inputs and three personnel injury inputs. Chapter Two breaks down the costs of different rescue capabilities. Chapter Three describes the rescue capability inputs—the MTFs, air assets, and airfields—that currently exist in Africa. The MTFs include DoD MTFs, allied (British, French, German, and Italian) MTFs, and, potentially, host-nation hospitals.

Chapter Four describes the personnel injury inputs of PAR, survival curves, and mortality risk distributions. PAR includes DoD and other U.S. government personnel assigned to Africa. The survival curves are drawn from the military medical literature, while the mortality risk distributions are drawn from the historical combat record. Chapter Four details the methodology by which we use these data to construct survivability timelines.

Chapter Five discusses two outputs from the rescue model: optimal rescue paths and optimal asset-location pairings. The optimal rescue paths are the most direct routes to the highest possible levels of medical care. The optimal asset-location pairings are the best marginal investments in rescue capabilities. To reiterate, each additional rescue asset represents an investment in one of the following options: a pair (or "node") of fixed-wing aircraft, a pair (or "node") of rotary-wing aircraft, a fixed DCS unit, or a mobile DCS unit. Each additional investment option is paired with an airfield location, resulting in a succession of optimal asset-location pairings, in order of diminishing marginal cost-effectiveness. Chapter Five concludes with a discussion of the key findings from the cost-effectiveness comparisons. Based on these findings, Chapter Six offers our recommendations for improving rescue in Africa over the long term.

CHAPTER TWO

Cost Analysis of Rescue Asset Options

As noted in Chapter One, AFRICOM's rescue requirements are unique, because its mission and operational environment do not correspond to the traditional template of other geographic combatant command theaters. The limited scale yet widely distributed nature of AFRICOM's operations, its semipermissive security conditions across key operational areas, and the ambiguities of kinetic activity outside declared theaters of active armed conflict (ODTAAC) all combine to create rescue requirements in AFRICOM that do not conform neatly to joint doctrine or the assumptions implicit in DoD's processes for joint operational planning, capability development, and global force management.

A primary implication of this uniqueness is that the capabilities best suited to fulfilling AFRICOM's rescue requirements are themselves unique. DoD's existing force structure contains, for example, no organization that is deliberately organized, trained, and equipped to sustain multiple small-scale DCS teams on a steady-state basis in austere, semipermissive locations at extended distances from supporting infrastructure. By *DCS teams*, we refer to both fixed DCS teams (those that have injured personnel transported to them) and mobile DCS teams (those that are moved to injured personnel). In practice, both kinds of DCS capabilities have been approximated in an ad hoc fashion by utilizing elements of defense organizations and private contractors created primarily for other purposes. But in joint doctrine, there is no agreed-upon label for the capability of DCS teams, partly because it encompasses elements of PR, CASEVAC, MEDEVAC, and AE. Likewise, there is no standard design for a DCS capability in the domains of joint operational planning, joint or service capability development, or global force management.

As a result of the uniqueness of AFRICOM rescue capabilities, we were not able to obtain reliable cost estimates of these capabilities. Given these challenges, this chapter presents our cost-estimating approach and findings.

Cost Analysis Approach

To establish a basis for comparing the resource implications of alternative investments in rescue assets, we use commercial analogies to derive what we call a *commercial-equivalent cost estimate*.[1] This approach employs analogous commercial services as a basis for estimating the costs of a unique military capability, such as DCS teams, for which DoD cost estimates do not exist.[2]

There are at least two reasons to believe that the commercial analogies approach is appropriate in this case. First, there are commercial entities that offer aviation and DCS capabilities analogous to those required to meet AFRICOM rescue requirements. These entities routinely work with DoD, U.S. government, and United Nations elements to provide steady-state capabilities in austere conditions, including in Africa. As a result, not only do these commercial entities represent useful organizational analogs, but two variations of the entities—contractor-owned, contractor-operated companies and/or contractor-owned, government-operated companies—may themselves be viable solutions to DoD's aviation and DCS requirements. Cost data from these entities are therefore both directly and indirectly useful to our analysis.

Second, commercial entities offering this capability employ analogous inputs to those that would be employed by military organizations possessing these capabilities. The surgical team capabilities required for a rescue mission would be identical regardless of whether the mission is manned by uniformed personnel or by contractors. Much the same can be said for the aircrew and support personnel for an aircraft. And, of course, the machines themselves may be indistinguishable. From an economic perspective, the cost structure for both types of entities ought to be similar.[3] DoD may have to pay a premium to attract personnel to the colors, who can then be ordered to deploy at any time and are subject to the Uniform Code of Military Justice. But this premium is offset on the commercial side by the need for a profit margin to attract capital.

Aircraft Airlift: Fixed-Wing or Rotary-Wing

To inform our analysis of aircraft costs, we reviewed recent DoD contracts for commercial airlift service providers operating in Africa as well as responses to a 2016 U.S. Spe-

---

[1]   In most cases, we find that the results are insensitive to the relative costs; however, with both shorter alert times and mobile DCS, the effectiveness of additional DCS and aircraft are comparable, and hence the cost could be a differentiating factor.

[2]   We use the term *DCS* to emphasize that these teams are smaller and more mobile—focused on damage control surgery as opposed to surgery more broadly—than the forward surgical teams (FSTs) or expeditionary medical support (EMEDS) teams deployed during OEF and OIF.

[3]   For an overview, see Cusumano (2016). For a broader discussion of cost comparisons between DoD run military treatment facilities and private hospitals, see Lurie (2016).

cial Operations Command request for information (RFI) regarding industry capabilities to provide civilian-model rotary-wing aircraft to support special operations forces in Africa. Both types of information included the costs of establishing and sustaining contractor team encampments within the AFRICOM AOR and operating temporarily from forward, austere locations. While this approach is not a precise analog to providing airlift support to DCS teams, the missions are sufficiently similar for the cost data to provide meaningful insight.

One notable aspect of the available contract and RFI data is their high degree of variability. The estimated cost of contractor airlift in Africa varies widely across commercial entities as well as operating locations, mission sets, environments, and availabilities of support infrastructure. Our best data come from the rotary-wing contracts and cost estimates provided in response to U.S. Special Operations Command's RFI. But for both the light fixed-wing and the medium rotary-wing capabilities, the actual or estimated costs varied by approximately a factor of two.[4]

Moreover, based on this data, the commercial-equivalent cost estimate for a single airlift node of either two fixed-wing or two rotary-wing aircraft is more or less the same: approximately $10 million annually. But the data also show a significant range of cost in both cases—from $5 million to $20 million—depending on specifics beyond the scope of this work.

DCS Team: Fixed or Mobile

Estimating the cost of a forward-deployed, small-scale DCS team also proved challenging. We consulted representatives of one commercial entity that provides medical services to U.S. and UN personnel in contingency environments, including in Africa. These representatives developed a first-order cost estimate to inform our analysis. The basis for their estimate was a formal proposal for a directly analogous capability developed by the company for DoD a short time before we engaged with the company to discuss this analysis.

According to the company's estimate, the cost of attracting and sustaining a DCS team of about the same size as analogous DoD teams, such as U.S. Air Force SOSTs, would be approximately $3.5 million per year. This includes the cost of additional personnel to provide a rotation base of 1-to-1 (one team is deployed for each one that is not), alternating every six weeks. In addition, the cost of the medical materiel to equip and sustain the team would be approximately $5 million for initial procurement plus another $1 million annually thereafter to replace consumed and expired materiel.

---

[4]   U.S. Special Operations Command Request For Information H92222-16-R-NSRW, March 2016, U.S. Navy contract N00189-14-C-0056 to AAR Airlift Group, Inc., June 10, 2014; *Alion Science & Technology, Inc.* subcontract 1137617 to Erickson Helicopters, Inc., November 4, 2014; U.S. Transportation Command contract HTC711-13-D-C013 to Berry Aviation, Inc., July 25, 2013; Martin, 2013; Irish and Flynn, 2013.

When life support and other sustainment expenses are included, the representatives estimated that $10 million would be a reasonable scoping factor for a contract DCS team dealing with a low rate of seriously injured patients. Depending on the operating location, tempo, and other unpredictable factors, one of our interlocutors estimated that the cost might easily climb to $15 million per year.

To supplement this single estimate of $10 million per year from a potential commercial provider, we employed a "bottom-up build" approach to estimate the labor, travel, and material costs of a comparable civilian equivalent to an SOST or a U.S. Air Force mobile field surgical team (MFST).[5] We used data from the Bureau of Labor Statistics (Bureau of Labor Statistics, undated), an online salary survey service (Salary. com, undated), the U.S. Department of State (U.S. Department of State, undated), and other sources. However, a number of variables introduced significant uncertainty into the validity of our cost analysis, most notably the potential cost of incentivizing highly skilled and well-paid medical professionals to suspend their practices or medical industry careers to accept the challenge of operating a mobile surgical unit in the austere, potentially hostile environment that is central Africa.

Our bottom-up build suggests that the combined domestic salaries of a single, full-time, five- to six-person commercial DCS team equivalent to an MFST or SOST could be in the range of $1 million to $2 million annually, depending on the team size and composition (e.g., general surgeon versus trauma surgeon versus orthopedic surgeon). However, these costs are based on peacetime, routine work schedules (i.e., 40- to 50-hour work weeks) in the United States. State Department foreign service professionals who are posted to certain dangerous locations in Africa are eligible to receive hardship and danger pay bonuses amounting to as much as 70 percent on top of their regular salary compensation (U.S. Department of State, undated), suggesting that a civilian surgical team could command at least 1.7 times their normal salaries ($1.7 million to $3.4 million annually) for time spent in similar environments in Africa.

As our analysis shows, the expected patient throughput in AFRICOM is relatively low. The low levels of clinical activity, combined with the potentially austere clinical conditions at the African locations, would suggest a need to rotate multiple teams of civilian DCS personnel between home and theater on a regular basis to maintain their medical skills and certifications in peacetime hospitals or medical practice settings. Depending on the rotation schedule, a civilian DCS service provider would likely incur additional direct, indirect, and/or overhead costs for recruiting and maintaining multiple DCS teams as needed to provide DCS services to AFRICOM on a continuing or recurring basis. Based on the SOST experience, these teams would need a dwell-to-deploy ratio of at least 2-to-1 (not just 1-to-1, as cited in the single bid above). Moreover, an equivalent commercial provider would likely need to cover the

---

[5]   Although SOSTs and MFSTs are examples of DCS teams, they remain difficult for costing purposes because of the complex nature of DoD's medical community and accounting policies.

costs of these multiple teams while they maintain their skills in domestic trauma centers. This 3-to-get-1 requirement would increase the potential salary costs to $5.1 million to $10.2 million.

In addition to the salary costs, a commercial DCS provider would need to incur the rotation costs of transporting personnel to and from Africa, as well as the billeting, meal, and other incidental expenses associated with overseas deployments. These costs could vary greatly depending on deployment locations and conditions. If, for instance, a deployed civilian DCS team were co-located with a military unit and were provided lodging, meals, and other services by the government, the costs might be relatively low—perhaps tens of thousands of dollars each year. If, however, the DCS team were deployed completely "on the economy," the cost of lodging, meals, and incidental expenses for the deployed civilian DCS team could be in the range of $400,000 to $700,000 per year, depending on the locations and negotiated per diem rates.[6]

Finally, a commercial provider of DCS teams would also incur the costs to procure, maintain, and replenish the medical equipment and supplies used by those teams. Once again, the costs of equipment and supplies could fall across a wide range, depending on the nature of the work performed and the conditions or infrastructure at the deployed locations. If a deployed civilian DCS team had access to, or were supported by, the U.S. government or military medical infrastructure (e.g., Class VIII supplies), the material costs could be relatively low. If, on the other hand, material were needed to establish a deployed civilian DCS capability from a cold start, the initial equipment costs could range as high as single-digit millions of dollars, with annual maintenance or replenishment costs thereafter on the order of a few hundred thousand to potentially 1 million dollars per year (Naval Health Research Center, undated; commercial provider interview).

The bottom-up build therefore produces a similarly wide range of potential cost estimates. In this case, the estimates add up to $6 million to $12 million per year, depending on a large number of unpredictable factors.

It is important to underscore that all of the cost categories discussed in both of the cost-estimating approaches above—the salaries, rotations, deployments, and supplies—would apply to both fixed and mobile DCS teams. For a mobile DCS team to move to the patient's location, it would generally need to do so by aircraft, but the aircraft costs are accounted for separately from the DCS team cost. Thus, if an operating location had both a new mobile DCS team and a new pair of aircraft dedicated to rescue missions, there would be two new rescue assets in total, each costing about $10 million, for a total approximate cost of $20 million annually. On the other hand, some existing DCS teams, assuming appropriate training, could be made mobile with

---

[6]   Per diem calculations based on (1) authors' informal internet survey of commercial hotel costs in representative locations throughout the central Africa region and (2) fiscal year (FY) 2017 DoD per diem rates as extracted from the website of the Defense Travel Management Office (undated).

the addition of alert aircraft, or some existing alert aircraft could be combined with additional DCS teams with appropriate training.

Cost Summaries

Given the uncertainty in our cost estimations, we use a round scoping factor of $10 million as an annual cost estimate for each of the four alternative components of a rescue capability: the fixed-wing airlift node, the rotary-wing airlift node, the fixed DCS team, or the mobile DCS team. In all four cases, the annual marginal cost would be roughly $10 million, with potential costs ranging from $5 million to $20 million per year.

Although each of the four alternative components would play a distinct role in enhancing AFRICOM's rescue capabilities, within a very broad range of uncertainty the cost of each component could be comparable. Because of the approximate similarity of costs across the four investment options, we simplify the cost-effectiveness analysis to come, reducing it to an analysis of effectiveness.

CHAPTER THREE

"Rescue Capability" Inputs

The first three effectiveness variables in the rescue model consist of "rescue capability" inputs. These represent the rescue resources that currently exist in Africa or could be added there. The inputs include MTFs, air assets, and airfields. This chapter discusses each input but focuses on MTFs as well as host-nation hospitals that could potentially complement MTFs.

Medical Treatment Facilities

MTFs currently available for rescued personnel across AFRICOM, including in Europe, fall into two categories: a "role 2" facility can perform DCS, while a "role 4" facility is a definitive care hospital in Germany.

Broadly speaking, medical professionals in AFRICOM perform two categories of medical care that are pertinent to rescue missions in Africa: first responder care and DCS.[1] In general, first responder care is the only category of care initially available to injured personnel in the field, whereas DCS is available once either the injured personnel is moved to an available MTF, or a DCS team moves to the patient. We distinguish between the two levels of care in greater detail below.

First Responder Care

When a person is injured in the field, initial care will be delivered either by the injured person or by other personnel. In joint doctrine (JP 4-02, 2012), this initial care consists of "role 1" care; however, the Joint Medical Planning Tool (JMPT) divides role 1 care into four tiers because of the range of capabilities of role 1 care providers. These

---

[1] First responder care and DCS encompass five of the seven roles of care in the U.S. military's Joint Medical Planning Tool (JMPT) (Teledyne Brown Engineering, Inc., 2015), as will be explained in Chapter Four. We consolidate some roles to distinguish more clearly between the levels of care associated with rescue missions and thus to enhance the analytical precision of our model.

providers range from the patients themselves or their fellow team members rendering immediate assistance (self-aid/buddy care); to combat medics; to battalion aid stations, which are staffed by physician assistants or physicians; to Navy/Marine Corps shock trauma platoons, which have larger teams of emergency medicine physicians and other care providers. The JMPT distinguishes among these levels of care based on the roles of the providers, designating self-aid/buddy care as role 1, combat medic care as role 1A, battalion aid station care as role 1B, and shock trauma platoon care as role 1C.

For purposes of our model, we assume that injured personnel in need of rescue will quickly receive a fairly similar level of emergency care from their unit's medical provider—whether that be a physician, physician assistant, independent duty corpsman, or 18D special operations medic—and that the abilities of these providers to deliver this kind of care in these types of circumstances will be equivalent to role 1B care as defined in the JMPT. For further simplicity of analysis and exposition, we will hereafter refer to any such emergency care administered by any category of provider as simply *role 1 care* or *first responder care*.

Damage Control Surgery

Severely injured trauma patients will often require care beyond that which can be provided in the field by any category of provider. This additional care could include surgical interventions to stop bleeding, restore circulation, or relieve pressure. In the JMPT and in joint doctrine (JP 4-02, 2012), this next level of care is known as *role 2 care* or *forward resuscitative surgery*. However, in keeping with AFRICOM's terminology and to emphasize the relatively limited level of surgical interventions, we refer to this level of care as *damage control surgery* (DCS).[2] We believe that DCS is more descriptive of both the intent and the limitations of surgical care that a patient may expect to receive in an austere environment.

To reiterate, we consider two types of DCS: fixed and mobile. We examine the effects of both. As we envision them, both types of DCS teams would be considered by joint doctrine to be "role 2 light maneuver" (2LM) in that they would be light, easily relocated, and "able to conduct advanced resuscitation procedures up to damage control surgery" (JP 4-02, 2012). Neither the fixed nor mobile DCS teams would be "role 2 enhanced" (role 2E), because they would not have a formal intensive care unit or ward beds. (We recognize that certain existing capabilities in theater might be considered role 2E, and that role 2E facilities can certainly perform DCS.)

The difference between fixed and mobile in our analysis lies primarily in the concepts of operation. With fixed DCS, patients are brought to a DCS location to receive

---

[2] The capabilities of a DCS team would be significantly less than a role 2 FST or EMEDS, particularly when operating in austere environments.

care. This follows the traditional model of a patient being transported to surgical care and then moved by an en route asset to a higher echelon of care. With mobile DCS, the team would move to the patient's location, perform the necessary stabilizing surgery on site (whether in a shelter of opportunity or in the back of a parked aircraft), and provide en route care as the patient is transported to the next destination. The mobile DCS teams are trained to provide ongoing patient management until arriving at a higher level of care.

One example of a fixed DCS capability is the MFST. As the initial surgical team that is deployed to an airbase as it is opened, an MFST consists of a general surgeon, an orthopedic surgeon, an anesthesia provider, an emergency medicine physician, and an operating room nurse or technician (Carlton and Pilcher, 1997). Another example is the SOST, a U.S. Air Force capability that evolved from the MFST concept to better support special operations (Ervin, 2008). Army FSTs or Navy/Marine Corps forward resuscitative surgical systems can also provide fixed DCS capabilities. The Army and Navy/Marine Corps teams are larger, although efforts are under way to create smaller versions of them.

An example of a mobile DCS capability was the U.S. Air Force's Tactical Critical Care Evacuation Team—Enhanced (TCCET-E). The TCCET-E consisted of a surgeon, an anesthesia provider, an emergency medicine physician, a critical care nurse, and an operating room technician. TCCET-E teams traveled aboard C-17 or C-130 AE flights to patient locations; performed surgery on the ground or, if absolutely necessary, in the air; and then provided en route care as the patient was evacuated to higher echelons of care. (As of March 2017, the Air Force was in the process of revising both the MFST and TCCET-E concepts into a new and integrated austere surgical team concept that would have ground-based and air-mobile versions, respectively, and that would differ only in some additional training for the air-mobile version.)

Host-Nation Hospitals

We collected data on the medical capabilities and limitations of host-nation hospitals in the AFRICOM AOR. Regarding the medical capabilities of these hospitals, we analyzed data from their respective medical verification organizations and reconciled these data with findings from the U.S. intelligence community and U.S. State Department. Regarding the medical limitations of these hospitals, we investigated the safety of the blood supply across Africa and assessed the implications for relying on host-nation facilities in AFRICOM force planning.

Verification of Host-Nation Capabilities

We sought to identify host-nation hospitals that could offer the equivalent of DCS care, requiring us to define a consistent threshold for such a capability (JP 4-02, 2012,

p. III-2). Using State Department data, we started with a list of 160 facilities that offer a surgical, preferably trauma, capability at an inpatient hospital with an operating room (U.S. Department of State, Bureau of Consular Affairs, undated). The State Department cautions, though, that it is "not responsible or liable for the professional ability or quality of service you may receive from a doctor or hospital on a list" (U.S. Department of State, Bureau of Consular Affairs, undated). Therefore, the State Department's list cannot serve as a credible indicator of medical capabilities but merely as a listing of available resources.

Given the State Department's data limitations and associated caveats, we gathered data from three medical verification organizations that have evaluated hospitals in Africa:

- International SOS Government Services, Inc. (International SOS), which is also the private evaluation contractor for DoD's TRICARE Overseas Program (TOP)
- Joint Commission International (JCI)
- Trauma Society of South Africa (TSSA).[3]

Figure 3.1 shows 19 African cities in which host-nation hospitals were evaluated and verified by International SOS or JCI. (The two TSSA locations, in the vicinity of Johannesburg, South Africa, are not visible on the map.) In total, 32 hospitals were verified by these organizations across the 20 African cities. Several of the hospitals were verified by two of the organizations. The map differentiates between two types of host-nation facilities evaluated by International SOS: those affiliated with DoD's TOP (represented by solid green dots) and those not affiliated with TOP (represented by hollow green dots).

One of the benefits of DoD's TOP is called Prime Remote; it covers the health-care expenses for active-duty service members and their eligible dependents in remote locations around the world (TRICARE, 2016). The contracts of TOP's Prime Remote health care providers require them to provide inpatient care on a cashless claim basis, meaning that TRICARE settles the bills directly with the providers, reducing the burden on DoD personnel receiving care. Such coverage benefits do not apply to service members and their dependents for care delivered at non-TOP hospitals (comparable to "out-of-network" hospitals in stateside health insurance programs).

The Defense Health Agency (DHA) awarded TOP's evaluation contract to International SOS in September 2015 (International SOS, 2013). International SOS evaluators visit TOP's Prime Remote hospitals in Africa every three years to evaluate them for TRICARE. These evaluations are based on host-nation standards rather than U.S.

---

[3]   We use the term *verification* rather than *accreditation*, because International SOS does not examine and vet facilities to the level of accreditation.

Figure 3.1
Host-Nation Hospital Sites and Verification Sources

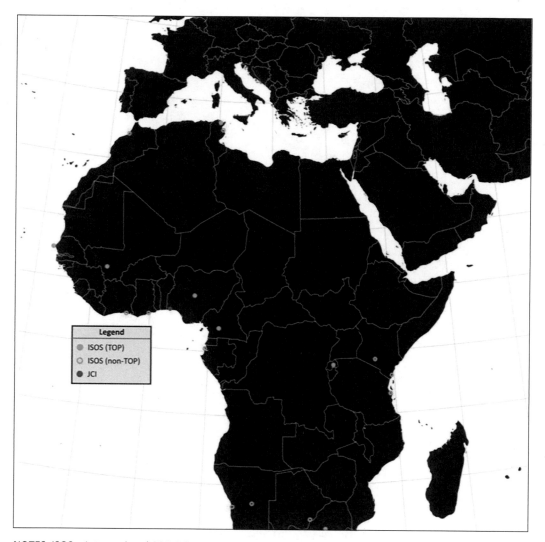

NOTES: ISOS = International SOS; TOP = TRICARE Overseas Program; JCI = Joint Commission International.

standards. As a result, the quality of Prime Remote hospitals across Africa fluctuates by country.

Beyond serving as the evaluator of many TOP and non-TOP facilities through-out Africa, International SOS provides medical services to more than 10,000 clients, including multinational companies, nongovernmental organizations, and government institutions (International SOS, 2017). The medical contractor has established a global network of its own clinics, which provide a standardized level of modern medical care.[4]

Due to this scope and experience, International SOS has a well-established methodology for verifying medical capabilities around the world. Its verification system was developed over several years through collaboration between International SOS medical teams and Global Assistance Network experts.[5] Those conducting International SOS site visits include physicians, nurses, aviation specialists, and security staff. The aggregated International SOS data on hospitals within the AFRICOM AOR show that all 32 facilities evaluated by International SOS in Africa meet the requisite medical capability for our definition of surgical care.[6]

The second verification organization, JCI, is a worldwide, not-for-profit accreditation agency. Established in 1994 and now active in more than 100 countries, JCI has accredited more than 800 facilities (Joint Commission, 2016). JCI's approval signifies that a facility has passed an independent assessment of international health care standards and is deemed of international quality.[7] JCI accreditation is recognized by International SOS and several other medical institutions, including the World Health Organization (WHO). In August 2005, WHO designated JCI as a WHO Collaborating Center on Patient Safety Solutions (World Health Organization, 2005). We identify three JCI-accredited hospitals that are capable of surgical medical care in the AFRICOM AOR.

The final verification organization is TSSA, an independent accreditation agency in South Africa. Affiliated with the South African Medical Association and the Association of Surgeons of South Africa, TSSA assigns accredited trauma units throughout the country one of three ratings, from level one for life-threatening injuries down to level three for minor injuries. Given the nature of injuries considered in this study, we include in our list of DCS-capable hospitals those that score either a level one or a level two within the TSSA accreditation scheme. There are five such hospitals, and all are located in the vicinity of Johannesburg (Trauma Society of South Africa, 2017).

After eliminating duplications in the data from the three organizations, we ended up with a list of 32 distinct host-nation hospitals, spanning 20 cities and 15 countries that are capable of DCS surgical care in the AFRICOM AOR. We reconciled these findings with those from the National Center for Medical Intelligence (NCMI) and the State Department. NCMI, an element of the Defense Intelligence Agency, gathers

---

[4]   The International SOS clinics typically result from client activity in a remote region, such as the operation of hydrocarbon facilities in the Sahara Desert.

[5]   The Global Assistance Network is a service of AXA Assistance, a private company offering travel assistance.

[6]   Some TOP Prime Remote sites differ from those recommended by International SOS to other clients. This can possibly be explained by the existence of International SOS contractual arrangements designed exclusively for active-duty service members seeking care.

[7]   These standards are published in Joint Commission International (2014).

intelligence on medical issues related to foreign militaries and to operating environments throughout the world (NCMI, undated). NCMI also publishes health system infrastructure assessments for several countries in Africa; these assessments include lists of recommended medical facilities for DoD personnel and U.S. citizens. The NCMI-recommended facilities were consistent with the 32 hospitals approved by the verification organizations.

As for the State Department literature, we collected the emergency action plans (EAPs) from all U.S. embassies in the AFRICOM AOR.[8] Similar to the NCMI infrastructure assessments, the State Department EAPs recommend host-nation medical facilities for U.S. government personnel and their dependents. The EAP-recommended facilities similarly matched the host-nation hospitals approved by the three verification organizations. In sum, through an amalgamation of private, not-for-profit, and government vetting sources, we found that 32 host-nation hospitals in Africa have the requisite surgical capabilities to serve as DCS facilities.

Medical Limitations in Africa

Although we assessed that 32 hospitals in Africa have adequate surgical capabilities, there is an extremely important caveat with respect to the safety of the blood supply throughout the continent. It is widely acknowledged that blood transfusions throughout Africa pose a very significant risk of transmitting an infectious disease.

In a 2009 comparative cross-country research study, it was estimated that the median risks of acquiring human immunodeficiency virus (HIV), hematopoietic necrosis virus (HNV), or hepatitis C virus (HCV) from a single unit of blood in sub-Saharan Africa were 1, 4.3, and 2.5 infections per 1,000 units, respectively (Jayaraman et al., 2010). In other words, the odds of not contracting HIV, HNV, or HCV from a single unit of transfused blood in sub-Saharan Africa were estimated to be 99.9 percent, 99.57 percent, and 99.75 percent, respectively. Thus, the odds of not contracting any of these infections from a single unit of blood would be $0.999 \times 0.9957 \times 0.9975 = 0.9922$, or 99.22 percent. However, based on the U.S. military's Technical Manual TM 8-227-12 (2011), we estimate that a trauma patient would need to receive, on average, six units of blood. This would translate to cumulative odds of not contracting any of the three viruses from six units of blood to be $(0.9922)^6 = 0.954$, or 95.4 percent. Conversely, the cumulative risk of a trauma patient receiving blood infected with HIV, HNV, and/or HCV in sub-Saharan Africa would be 4.6 percent—or roughly one out of every 22 trauma patients treated. It is not surprising that DHA, International SOS, and NCMI strongly discourage the receipt of blood transfusions on the continent unless the situation is life-threatening and no other viable option is available.

The widespread challenges associated with the blood supply in Africa can be seen in NCMI's country-by-country blood safety index (NCMI, 2017). The index rates

---

[8]   The U.S. Embassy EAPs are not available to the general public.

the safety of the blood supply in each country as excellent, good, fair, poor, or unsuitable, based on various intelligence metrics. According to NCMI, the vast majority of countries in the AFRICOM AOR receive a rating of poor or unsuitable, and only eight receive a rating of fair, with zero rated as good or excellent for its blood safety. Even South Africa does not have what is deemed a fully safe blood supply, because the country does not conduct Food and Drug Administration–required testing for human T-lymphotropic virus (HTLV) I and II antibodies on collected blood. Moreover, the country experiences frequent blood shortages. Figure 3.2 illustrates the NCMI ratings of overall health care capabilities (beyond blood safety) across Africa, but these overall ratings are largely consistent with the NCMI blood supply ratings.

In summary, whereas the surgical capabilities of 32 hospitals across Africa appear to meet the requisite DoD standard for providing surgical care, the safety of the blood supply in these hospitals poses a pervasive risk. Consequently, we assume that DoD will not rely on host-nation facilities for force planning purposes. But even though the blood safety hazard makes host-nation hospitals unacceptable for force planning purposes, there is still the possibility of utilizing host-nation hospitals when no other trauma care option is available. In such *in extremis* situations, the risk of contaminated blood may be less than the risk of delaying medical care.

Air Assets (Aircraft)

We took inventory of the air assets that are now potentially available from these locations for PR and CASEVAC missions throughout the AFRICOM AOR.[9] This inventory includes assets that are either dedicated (their primary mission is PR, and they are on alert for PR missions) or nondedicated (their primary mission is not PR, but they could perform PR missions). Dedicated U.S. assets were modeled on N+3 hours (they can launch a recovery within three hours of notice). We model all nondedicated U.S. assets, which by definition are not on alert, as being available on N+12 hours. As for allied aircraft, we use their stated alert times. We do not include redundant and lesser aircraft.

Airfields

In addition to the various AFRICOM basing locations, we account for the other potentially available civil and military airfields and their varying capacities throughout

---

[9] We use the term *potentially available* because some of these assets are not dedicated assets and therefore may be conducting other missions at the time they are needed.

Figure 3.2
Health Care Capabilities Across Africa

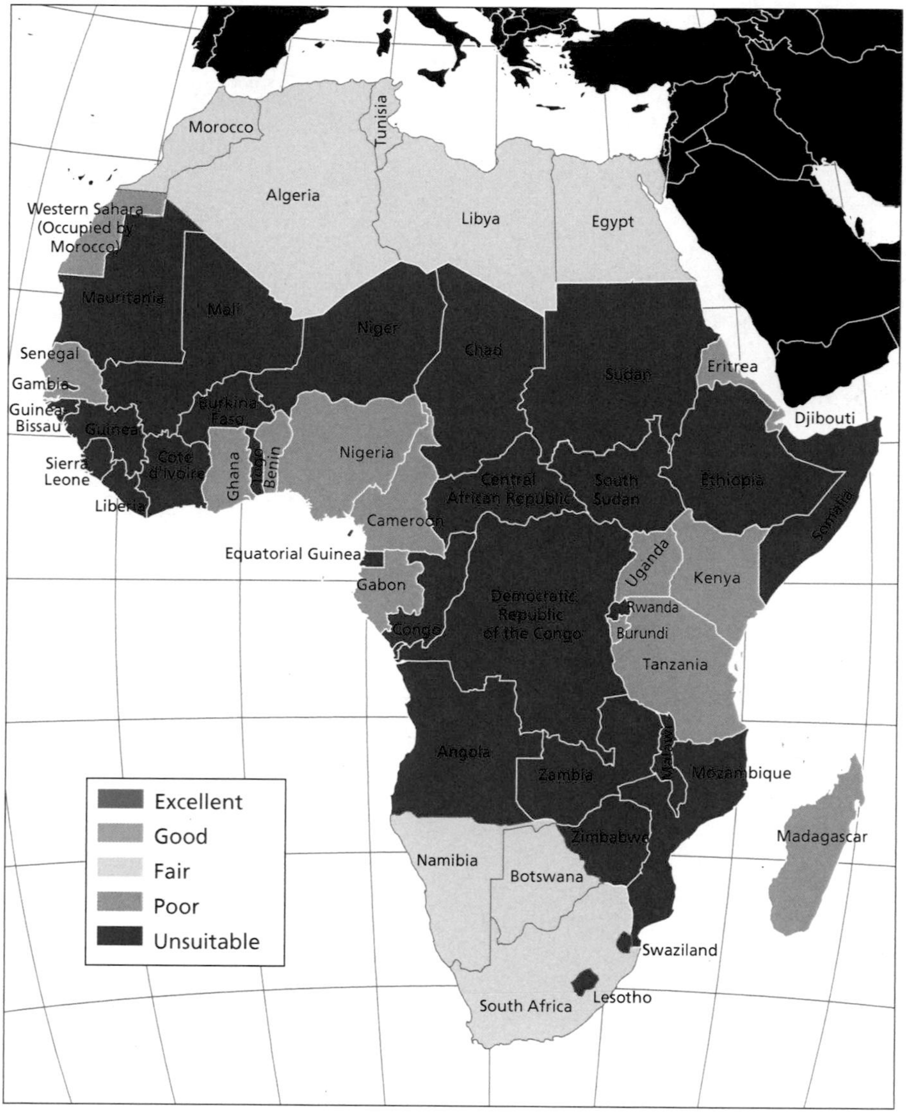

SOURCE: National Center for Medical Intelligence.
RAND RR2161z1-3.2

Africa. Thus, we add to our list of "rescue capability" inputs those African airfields that are contained within the Automated Air Facilities Information File (AAFIF).

We rate all of the airfields on the continent—including U.S., allied, and host-nation airfields—by maximum demonstrated capability. The most capable airfields can accommodate C-17 cargo planes. The intermediate airfields can accommodate C-130 turboprop planes. The least capable airfields can accommodate small fixed-wing and medium fixed-wing aircraft, examples of which are C-145 and C-146 twin-engine aircraft, B-350 turboprop planes, and U-28s.[10] As for airfields outside of Africa, we consider only the global mobility hubs. Figure 3.3 shows the ratings for the AFRICOM and all other potentially available airfields. In the map legend, the B-350 represents small fixed-wing and medium fixed-wing aircraft.

Full Inventory of Rescue Capability Inputs

In total, the baseline AFRICOM rescue capability inputs for our model include MTF locations, basing locations with air assets, and hundreds of airfields of varying maximum demonstrated capabilities. In addition, 32 host-nation hospitals in 20 African cities across 15 countries could be utilized for trauma care when no such care could otherwise be provided by U.S. or allied MTFs.

---

[10]   Higher-fidelity distinctions can be made between airfields and the aircraft they can support, but, for the purposes of comparing our investment options, such a distinction was not necessary.

Figure 3.3
Airfields by Maximum Demonstrated Capability

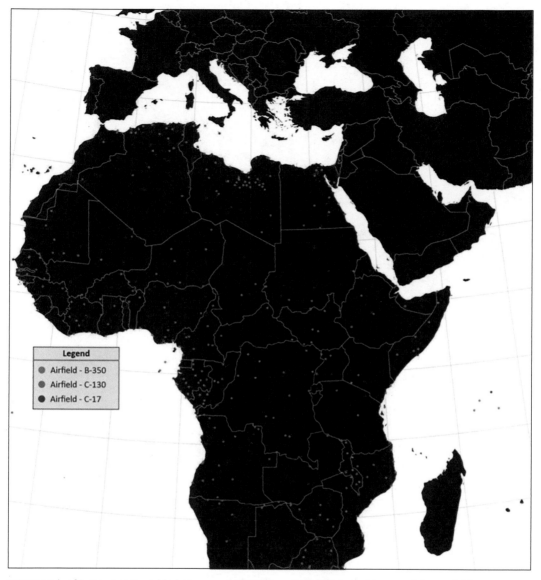

NOTE: Lack of instruments and lighting capabilities at some airfields could cause delays, which were not factored into the rescue model.

RAND *RR2161z1-3.3*

CHAPTER FOUR

"Personnel Injury" Inputs

The other trio of effectiveness variables in our rescue model consists of "personnel injury" inputs. These include PAR, survival curves, and mortality risk distributions. This chapter describes the PAR in Africa and then walks through our method of constructing average survival timelines, which establish the expected survival rates over time for personnel receiving different levels of care for different severities of life-threatening injuries. The timelines depend on preexisting data for survival curves and mortality risk distributions. Because the survival data are broken down by the levels of risk encountered, our initial survival timelines are also broken down by the levels of risk encountered. We then average the timelines across the levels of mortality risk and across the historical mortality risk distributions, allowing us to isolate the differences in expected survival rates based on response times and levels of care received. The chapter concludes with a discussion of PR data specific to AFRICOM, which show that PR events have been increasing and also extending beyond the AFRICOM AOR.

Population at Risk

The first "personnel injury" input is the total PAR. Figure 4.1 shows roughly where U.S. military personnel might be located in the AFRICOM AOR. The geographic dispersion of the PAR is a very significant factor in the model, as it influences not only the location of rescue assets but also the type of assets. For example, many small pockets of personnel at locations without an airfield would necessitate helicopters and mobile surgical teams, whereas a limited number of locations with large numbers of personnel would be best served by co-located surgical capabilities. Our exploration of additional assets and their respective locations will be discussed in Chapter Five.

Survival Data and Mortality Risk Distribution Data

The methodology used in this analysis to construct survivability timelines draws heavily from two data sources that are used widely in the defense medical community: the

Figure 4.1
Geographic Dispersion of Personnel Laydown

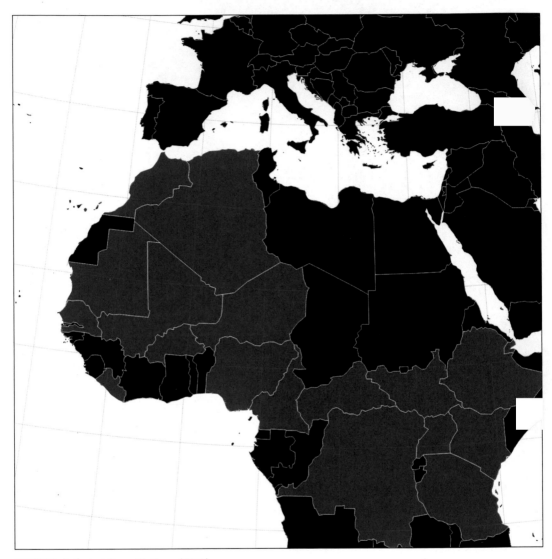

SOURCE: Adapted from McCann (2018).
RAND RR2161z1-4.1

Joint Medical Planning Tool (JMPT; Teledyne Brown Engineering, Inc., 2015) and the Medical Planners' Toolkit (MPTk; Naval Health Research Center, 2013).[1] The methodology draws on survival data from the JMPT and mortality risk distribution data from the MPTk.

---

[1]   We summarize this methodology here, but a more complete description can be found in two earlier RAND reports on this topic: Mouton and Godges (2016) and Mouton, Godges, and Chan (2018).

Survival Data from the JMPT

The second personnel injury input is a set of survival curves that vary according to the severity of injury suffered, the level of care administered, and the amount of time spent at each level of care (Mouton and Godges, 2016). To construct these survival curves, we first gather the survival data from the JMPT. Developed by the Naval Health Research Center and Teledyne Brown Engineering, the JMPT is the official medical planning tool of the DHA.

The JMPT assigns each injury type a condition code known as an ICD-9 code (ICD-9 stands for *International Classification of Diseases, 9th Revision*). There are more than 13,000 ICD-9 codes. The JMPT utilizes and incorporates more than 300 of the ICD-9 codes to cover the array of injuries that deployed military personnel are likely to encounter, ranging from tetanus to a closed fracture of nasal bones to an open head wound with complications.

The JMPT then matches each of its 300-plus condition codes to different probabilities of each condition resulting in one or as many as four mortality risk levels. Three of these risk levels indicate that the condition is life-threatening (with either a high, medium, or low mortality risk), while the fourth risk level indicates that the condition is non-life-threatening. Because the term *low mortality risk* might not adequately convey the seriousness of an injury that can kill someone, we refer to the JMPT's high, medium, and low mortality risk levels as mortality risks A, B, and C, respectively. All of them are potentially deadly.

Because each condition code can be assigned to no more than four mortality risk levels, it is the distribution among the four risks—and not the distribution among the hundreds of injuries or conditions—that we use in our mortality modeling. Thus, the model does not need to differentiate between such disparate wounds as "injury to kidney with open wound into cavity" and "open skull fracture without mention of [other] injury, unspecified state of consciousness," because both are modeled as having the same mortality risk (in this case, medium or B).

The JMPT also defines seven differentiated roles of care, in order of the increasing clinical sophistication associated with the actual roles played by medical care providers of increasing clinical sophistication. The seven JMPT roles are (1) self-aid/buddy care, (1A) first responder care, (1B) battalion aid station care, (1C) emergency trauma care, (2) forward resuscitative care, (3) theater hospitalization, and (4) definitive care (completion of recommended treatment). Prehospital care, commonly referred to as role 1, encompasses the four lower roles of care (1, 1A, 1B, and 1C). Hospital care encompasses the three higher roles of care (2, 3, and 4). Table 4.1 shows the prehospital and hospital roles as defined by the JMPT.

In creating the JMPT's simulation program, the Naval Health Research Center and Teledyne Brown Engineering constructed 28 survival curves, one for each pairing

Table 4.1
Prehospital and Hospital Roles of Care in the JMPT

Code	Level of Differentiated Care
1	Self- and buddy aid
1A	First response
1B	Aid station
1C	Emergency trauma care
2	Forward resuscitative care
3	Theater hospitalization
4	Definitive care

SOURCE: Teledyne Brown Engineering, Inc., 2015.

NOTE: When differentiating among different tiers of role 1 care, the JMPT uses the term *codes* to denote roles.

of four risk levels with seven care roles.[2] As one would expect, the higher the role of care received, the greater the likelihood of survival achieved. (As a patient progresses through one or more clinical steps toward higher roles of care, the mortality curve associated with each higher role affords the patient better odds of survival.)

As mentioned in Chapter Three, we revise the JMPT curves slightly for purposes of modeling and clarity. Specifically, we select the JMPT role 1B as the representative role of care that an injured person will initially receive in all cases. We rename this role 1B care as *role 1 care* or simply *first responder care*. For consistency with AFRICOM's terminology, we also replace the JMPT's *forward resuscitative care* with AFRICOM's *damage control surgery*, or DCS. We retain the terms of *theater hospital* and *definitive care* for roles 3 and 4, respectively. Table 4.2 shows the slightly revised roles and definitions of care that we use in this analysis.

The mortality risk levels and the medical care roles described above determine the survival curves and, by extension, the expected mortality rates along those curves. The JMPT survival curves were based either on expert opinion (for prehospital roles of care) or on medical records (for hospital roles of care).

For the prehospital roles of care ("first responder care" in our analysis), the curves were based on input from a panel of subject matter experts. The experts were asked, for example, "Out of 100 patients with a particular ICD-9 code, receiving only first responder care, how many of those 100 would you expect to survive a half hour after

---

2   In some cases, there is no mortality risk associated with an injury risk at a given level of care.

**Table 4.2
Revised Roles and Definitions of Care Used in
This Analysis**

Role	Definition of Care
1	First responder (18D/PA/MD)
2	Damage control surgery
3	Theater hospital
4	Definitive care

SOURCE: Teledyne Brown Engineering, Inc., 2015.
NOTE: 18D = Special Forces Medical Sergeant
(informally, special operations medic); PA =
physician's assistant; MD = medical doctor.

injury? Three hours?" The results were then fitted to Weibull curves showing the expected mortality rates as a function of time.

For patients receiving DCS and theater hospital care (roles 2 and 3), the JMPT survival curves were derived from patient data from OEF and OIF, covering about the first six or 24 hours post-injury, respectively. The results were then fitted to lognormal curves, producing the expected mortality rates as a function of time.

Figure 4.2 shows a simple binning of mortality risks for a range of ICD-9 codes, or patient conditions, based on expert input regarding the expected survival rates with first responder care alone. Conditions that fall on the higher end of the risk spectrum (and lower end of the survivability spectrum in the figure) include multisystem trauma involving injuries to the thorax, abdomen, head, spine, and major blood vessels. Conditions that fall on the lower end of the risk spectrum (and higher end of the survivability spectrum), yet are still life-threatening, include severe burns, traumatic amputations, pneumothoraxes (collapsed lungs), and hemothoraxes (accumulations of excess blood in the lungs). On the right side of the figure, the stacked red, yellow, and green column at hour 1 demarcates the expected survival boundaries for personnel with PCs that pose Mortality Risks A, B, and C, respectively.

As an example of the JMPT survival curves, Figure 4.3 shows the expected survival rates for injured personnel receiving only first responder care (role 1 care) for the three different levels of life-threatening injuries. The three curves in the figure show that, given first responder care alone, just 40 percent of personnel with life-threatening injuries posing a high mortality risk (Mortality Risk A) are expected to survive six hours after injury, whereas 66 percent of personnel with life-threatening injuries posing a medium mortality risk (Mortality Risk B) are expected to survive six hours, and 81 percent of personnel with life-threatening injuries posing a relatively 'low' mortality risk (Mortality Risk C) are expected to survive six hours. These and other JMPT survival curves represent the expected survival rates for patients only at a

Figure 4.2
JMPT Binning of ICD-9 Patient Conditions (PCs) Based on Mortality Risks

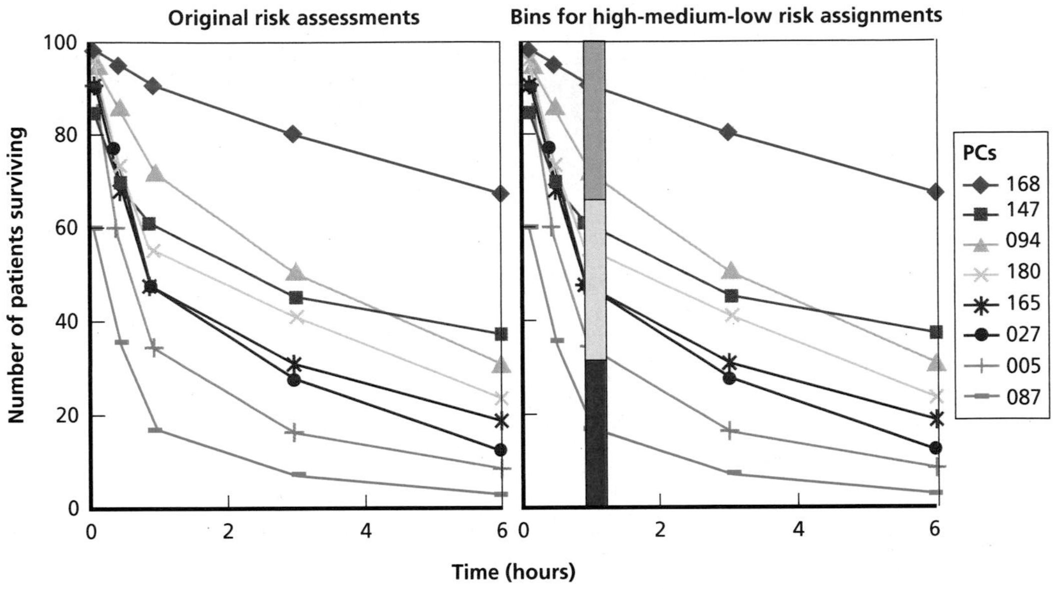

SOURCE: Adapted from Mitchell et al., 2004, Figure 9.
NOTES: JMPT versions up to 8.1 mapped each individual ICD-9 code (patient condition) to a single mortality risk, as shown by the red, yellow, and green column in the figure. In JMPT version 8.2, however, the methodology was improved to include probabilistically mapping each ICD-9 code to multiple mortality risk levels.
RAND *RR2161z1-4.2*

given care level—and not across the rescue chain, which typically involves ascending levels of care. As an injured person moves to higher levels of care, his or her expected survival rate will also shift upward onto higher survival curves associated with those higher levels of care. An example of such a composite curve will be provided later in this chapter.

Mortality Risk Distribution Data from the MPTk
The third and final personnel injury input is the historical distribution of injuries suffered at each mortality risk level. Combining the geographic distribution of the PAR with the survival curves and the historical mortality risk distributions allows us to predict the average percentage of injured personnel who will likely survive under varying 'rescue capability' conditions and time frames.

We consulted the MPTk, also developed by the Naval Health Research Center, for historical information about the mortality risk distributions of injuries suffered in combat zones. The MPTk uses the same 300-plus ICD-9 codes for patient conditions as specified in the JMPT. We used the MPTk distribution of mortality risk data across a sampling of historical military operations. In this way, both the military medical

Figure 4.3
JMPT Survival Curves with First Responder Care Alone (Role 1B)

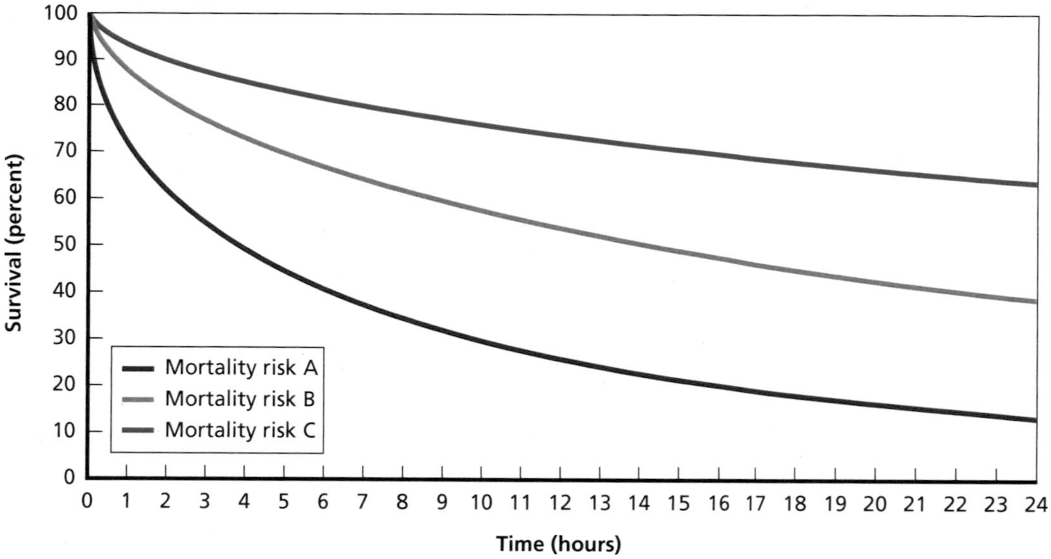

SOURCE: Teledyne Brown Engineering, Inc., 2015.
RAND *RR2161z1-4.3*

information on survival curves (from the JMPT) and the historical information on mortality risk distributions (from the MPTk) inform our findings about the average effects of different incident response speeds and capabilities on rescue missions. In other words, by combining the JMPT survival curves with the MPTk mortality risk distributions across historical events, we can plot the average expected relationships between survivability and time for personnel who suffer any types of life-threatening injuries. We can then isolate the effects of different response times and different levels of medical care received. Ultimately, this methodology will allow AFRICOM to focus on two key factors that it can actually control to some extent: incident response speed and medical care delivery.

For now, we focus on 15 historical MPTk datasets (Naval Health Research Center and Teledyne Brown Engineering, Inc., 2015). One of these datasets contains data from Africa (and another operation), and 13 of them contain data from OEF and OIF, beginning in 2001. The 15th includes historical information from Vietnam. We recognize that the available data may or may not be representative of the conditions that rescue missions are expected to face in Africa. But because very few rescue missions involving personnel with life-threatening injuries have recently been conducted in Africa, and because the known details about such missions are limited at any rate, constraining our dataset to Africa would offer insufficient data to conduct this analysis. Therefore, we rely on a collection of historical cases that represent a range of locations and conflict conditions. As it turns out, the results prove to be insensitive to the precise nature of each conflict. The 15 historical datasets we use for this analysis are as follows (in chronological order of start date):

- Vietnam (multiservice data on the conflict in Southeast Asia from 1965 to 1971)
- The Mayaguez Incident (the Khmer Rouge seizure of the SS *Mayaguez*, anchored offshore a Cambodian island, in May 1975) and Operation Gothic Serpent (the Battle of Mogadishu, Somalia, including the "Black Hawk Down" incident, from August to October 1993)
- OEF Air Force (U.S. Air Force data from Afghanistan, October 2001 to December 2014)
- OEF Army (U.S. Army data from Afghanistan, October 2001 to December 2014)
- OEF Marines (U.S. Marines data from Afghanistan, October 2001 to December 2014)
- OEF Navy (U.S. Navy data from Afghanistan, October 2001 to December 2014)
- OIF Air Force (U.S. Air Force data from Iraq, March 2003 to August 2010)
- OIF Army (U.S. Army data from Iraq, March 2003 to August 2010)
- OIF Marines (U.S. Marines data from Iraq, March 2003 to August 2010)
- OIF Navy (U.S. Navy data from Iraq, March 2003 to August 2010)
- OIF (multiservice data from Iraq, 2004 to 2009)
- OIF Second Battle of Fallujah (a joint American, Iraqi, and British offensive in Iraq, November and December 2004)
- OEF/OIF (multiservice data from Afghanistan and Iraq during the 2008/2009 surge in Iraq).
- OEF 2010 (multiservice data from Afghanistan for 2010)
- Operation New Dawn (operations in Iraq after the declared end of the OIF combat mission, 2010 and 2011).

Because the MPTk consolidated the Mayaguez Incident and Operation Gothic Serpent into a single dataset, called "raid," these two events appear as a combined case in our data as well, as shown in Table 4.3.

It is worth noting that the data in Table 4.3 do not represent the rate or frequency at which injuries might occur. Rather, the data represent the likely severity of an injury given that it has occurred. In addition, we are looking at injury severity only, not injury type. That is to say, even though the injuries experienced in Afghanistan and Iraq are likely to be very different from those potentially experienced in Africa, there is reason to believe that the distribution of severity may be similar, given the striking similarity of mortality risks across the historical datasets.

The consistency across historical events, ranging from Vietnam to recent conflicts, is highly suggestive of a certain level of invariance with respect to mortality risk distributions of life-threatening injuries. Figure 4.4 graphically shows this limited variation across the three mortality risk levels of interest. The mean likelihood of

Table 4.3
MPTk Historical Data Covering 15 Historical Events

Event	Non-Life-Threatening Injury	Life-Threatening Injury	Breakdown of Life-Threatening Injuries by Mortality Risk		
			Mortality Risk A	Mortality Risk B	Mortality Risk C
Vietnam (1965–1971)	66	34	25	27	48
Gothic Serpent/Mayaguez	77	23	30	26	44
OEF (Air Force)	77	23	25	25	50
OEF (Army)	79	21	24	26	50
OEF (Marine Corps)	75	25	29	26	45
OEF (Navy ashore)	75	25	23	26	51
OIF (Air Force)	77	23	22	23	55
OIF (Army)	76	24	25	24	51
OIF (Marine Corps)	77	23	32	24	44
OIF (Navy ashore)	75	25	27	25	48
OIF (2004–2009)	76	24	27	24	49
Second Battle of Fallujah	88	12	25	25	50
OEF/OIF (2008–2009)	77	23	23	25	53
OEF (2010)	77	23	26	26	48
New Dawn (2010–2011)	79	21	30	24	46
Average[a]	76	24	26	25	49
AFRICOM (FY16 update)	50	50	33	0	67

SOURCE: Naval Health Research Center and Teledyne Brown Engineering, Inc., 2016.
[a] To avoid double counting, the averages exclude New Dawn and OEF (2010), OEF (2008–2009), and Second Battle of Fallujah.

injured personnel facing a Mortality Risk A or a Mortality Risk B has each been about 25 percent, while the mean likelihood of injured personnel facing a Mortality Risk C has been nearly 50 percent. Moreover, the second and third quartiles in all three cases show that there has been very little divergence from those expected likelihoods across the historical datasets across the decades. Over the past 50 years, there has been very little change in the likelihood of injured personnel facing any of those mortality risk levels.

Figure 4.4
Consistency of MPTk Mortality Risk Estimates Across Historical Datasets

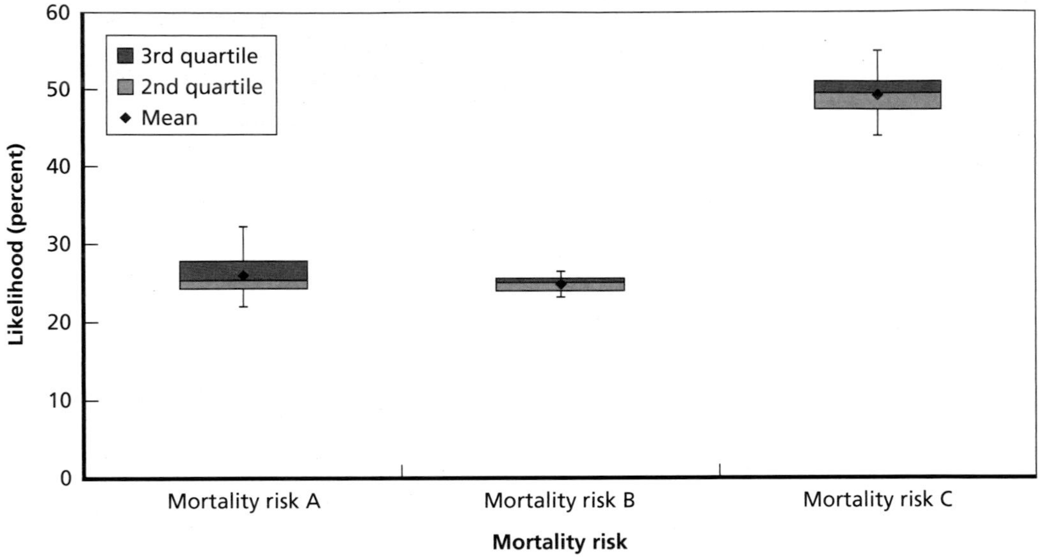

SOURCE: Naval Health Research Center and Teledyne Brown Engineering, Inc., 2016.
RAND *RR2161z1-4.4*

Averaging Across Risk Distributions

Once we exclude non-life-threatening injuries from our analysis (because they do not pose the same degree of urgency and thus are not particularly sensitive to any rescue posture), we can determine the average distribution of mortality risks across the 15 historical datasets, as specified at the bottom of Table 4.3 and as illustrated as the means in Figure 4.4. Based on that average distribution of mortality risks, we can then ascertain the weighted average survival rates across the 15 conflict scenarios (weighted by the historical average mortality risk distribution). The weighted average survival rates depend, of course, on the levels of care received by personnel facing the different mortality risks across the scenarios.

The weighted average survival rates for two different levels of care can be seen in the two survival curves in Figure 4.5. The lower curve is for first responder care; the higher curve is for DCS. Each curve shows the average expected survival rate, from hour to hour, for any patient with a life-threatening injury of any severity level receiving the specified care level in any of the 15 historical conflict scenarios or in any future conflict scenario.

As suggested above, patients will often advance from one role of care to the next. Patients may initially receive first responder care for six hours in the field and then receive DCS upon reaching a surgical facility. The expected survivability timeline for these patients will be a composite of the two role-of-care curves from Figure 4.5, as

Figure 4.5
Weighted Average Survival Curves, by Level of Care Received

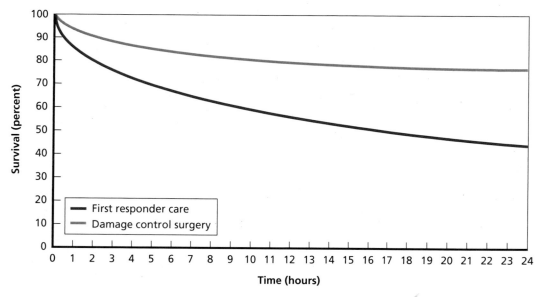

SOURCE: Teledyne Brown Engineering, Inc., 2015.
RAND RR2161z1-4.5

combined in Figure 4.6. In the latter case, the flatness of the DCS curve beginning at hour six replaces the steepness of the first responder curve as of that hour (although the DCS curve commences at a lower starting point than in Figure 4.5).[3]

---

[3]   A dashed continuation of role 1 care is shown in Figure 4.6 for reference.

Figure 4.6
Survival Curve for Those Receiving Role 1 Care, Then Role 2 Care

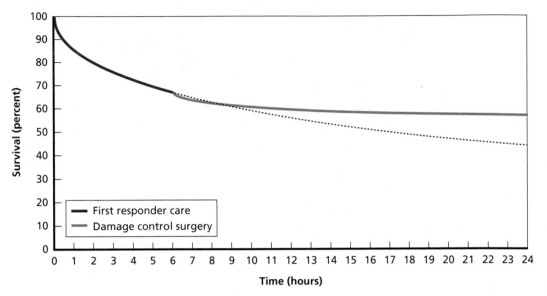

SOURCE: Teledyne Brown Engineering, Inc., 2015.

RAND RR2161z1-4.6

CHAPTER FIVE

Rescue Model Outputs

This chapter discusses two outputs from the rescue model: optimal rescue paths and optimal asset-location pairings. The optimal rescue paths are the most life-saving routes to higher levels of medical care. The optimal asset-location pairings are the best marginal investments in rescue capabilities. Each additional rescue asset represents an investment in one of the following: a pair (or node) of fixed-wing aircraft, a pair (or node) of rotary-wing aircraft, a fixed surgical unit, or a mobile surgical unit. These assets are treated independently—that is, an aircraft node does not imply any surgical capability, just as a surgical unit does not imply any aviation capability. In the model, each additional investment option is paired with an airfield location, resulting in a succession of optimal asset-location pairings, in order of diminishing marginal cost-effectiveness. The chapter concludes with a discussion of the key findings from the cost-effectiveness comparisons.

Optimal Rescue Paths

Our model charts alternative rescue paths as a first step toward estimating the survival rates that could be expected from different response speeds and care levels. For a given injury location and mortality risk, the model computes every possible combination of MTFs, air assets, and airfields that can be used for a rescue mission from that injury location and identifies the path with the maximum expected survival rate. The model also generates survival maps and computes the average statistics for incident response times, travel times to a DCS, and survival rates, depending on the mortality risks incurred.

The map in Figure 5.1 shows a purely notional case of an optimal rescue path identified by the rescue model for an individual injured in the Central African Republic. Even along this optimal path, the average survival rate for such an individual plummets quickly from 100 percent at the moment of injury (the expected survival rate always begins at 100 percent) to just 39.81 percent after 22 hours and 45 minutes of receiving first responder care (shown as role 1B care) en route to Obo. The expected survival rate falls further, to 35.74 percent, during the 4-hour, 37-minute flight to the

Figure 5.1
Optimal Rescue Path and Expected Survival (Notional)

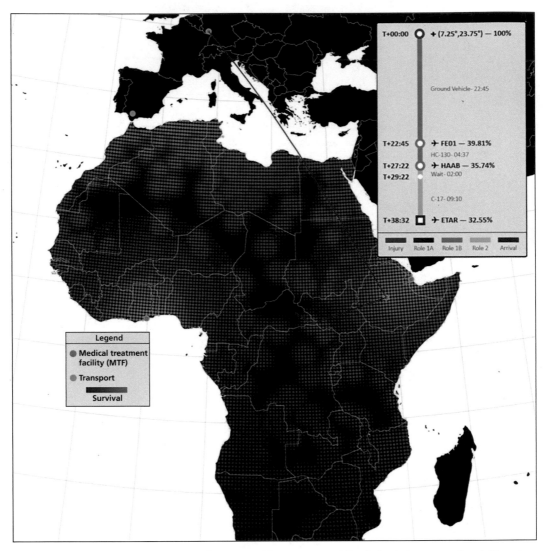

NOTES: FE01 = Boda Airport, Central African Republic; HAAB = Addis Ababa Bole International Airport, Ethiopia; ETAR - Ramstein Airport, Germany. Survival rates, MTFs, and transports displayed in the figure are notional and for illustrative purposes only.
RAND *RR2161z1-5.1*

role 2 facility, while the individual continues to receive first responder care. Finally, upon shifting to role 2 care and spending two hours in DCS, the patient continues on the role 2 curve aboard a C-17 flight to Ramstein, Germany, and the expected survival rate falls slowly to 32.55 percent over the next nine hours and ten minutes. By the time the individual reaches Landstuhl Regional Medical Center in Germany, more than 38 hours will have elapsed since the moment of injury.

The rescue model can run these computations to identify the optimal rescue path for any hypothetical individual injured anywhere in Africa—or, more precisely, in any Global Area Reference System (GARS) box on the continent. Each GARS box represents a 0.5-degree-by-0.5-degree plot of earth. There are approximately 10,000 such plots across the African continent.

The map in Figure 5.1 also shows each GARS box notionally shaded according to the average expected survival rate from that location. The model computes each rate based on the geographic location of the injury, the average survival timeline associated with the injury (as drawn from the JMPT), and the historical incidence of injury severity (as drawn from the MPTk). Each GARS box is shaded by its estimated survival rate, with the highest rates (brightest blue spots) often clustered around MTFs. In contrast, some of the darker (blacker) regions, including those in the middle of the continent, might be close to a transport site, but an aircrew would still need to travel a great distance to reach the transport site and then haul an injured person to the closest DCS team (as in the optimal rescue path charted above).

Optimal Asset-Location Pairings

The GARS map above serves as a point of departure for comparing the effects of alternative asset-location pairings that could raise the survival rates from rescue missions. It needs to be acknowledged that the survival rates cannot be raised drastically given the MTFs, air assets, and airfields currently available in AFRICOM.

To set the parameters of what is likely feasible, Figure 5.2 depicts a small "survival window" within two rescue posture extremes called "baseline risk" and "minimum risk." Baseline risk represents the current U.S. rescue posture in Africa. Minimum risk represents the estimated effect of unrealistically ambitious new investments in rescue capabilities, specifically the placement of a trio of assets, a DCS facility, an N+1 helicopter, and an N+6 C-17 plane—at more than 500 airfields across the AFRICOM AOR. As the figure shows, even this infeasible investment would raise the average expected survival rate for those with life-threatening injuries in Africa only 6.5 percentage points.

Because investing in all of the mitigations explored here at each of the airfields under consideration would likely be cost-prohibitive, we use the rescue model to identify the most cost-effective additional investment, or asset, paired with an airfield location, yielding the most cost-effective asset-location pairing at the margin. For each location, we assess the effectiveness and cost-effectiveness of these four investment options:

- light fixed-wing aircraft node (two airplanes)
- medium rotary-wing aircraft node (two helicopters)

Figure 5.2
Rescue Posture Gap, from Baseline to Ambitious Investments

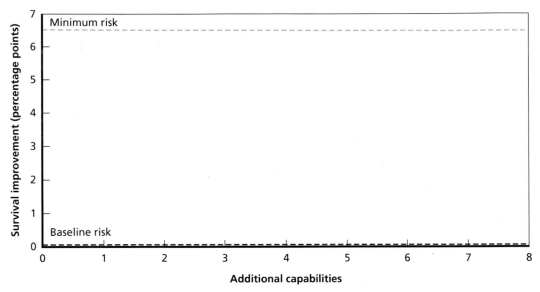

RAND *RR2161z1-5.2*

- "fixed" DCS team (a patient is moved to the DCS location)
- "mobile" DCS team (a DCS team can move to the patient location).[1]

As we presented in Chapter Two, the estimated cost of all four of the investment options at any of the locations is roughly identical, which simplifies our assessment of cost-effectiveness into an assessment of effectiveness. Based on previous AFRICOM contract data and on conversations with private contractors, the commercial-equivalent cost estimate for each of the four options—a light fixed-wing aircraft node, a medium rotary-wing aircraft node, a fixed DCS team, or a mobile DCS team—is about $10 million per year.[2]

We also consider decreasing the alert times of dedicated assets. We assume a standard alert time for aircraft of N+3. In the rescue model, we decrease the alert times for both the fixed-wing and the rotary-wing aircraft from the standard N+3 to N+1.[3]

---

[1]   Although a fixed DCS team can be relocated, its surgical capability cannot be moved quickly enough in response to a medical emergency. In contrast, a mobile DCS team can perform surgery at the patient's location and then move the patient as needed.

[2]   Additional training would be required for a DCS team to become mobile and to provide en route care. Because we assessed this to be a relatively small marginal cost, it was not explicitly incorporated into our cost analysis, but it is an important factor to consider.

[3]   Decreasing the alert times would naturally increase the cost of the assets. Based on conversations with contractors, the additional cost is estimated at 20 percent—or $2 million per year. Again, though, because of the

The rescue model calculates the marginal effectiveness, in terms of raising the expected survival rate, investing in each of the four assets, and using either aircraft alert time at all locations. Figure 5.3 illustrates the iterative nature of the methodology in comparing a succession of marginal results across the spectrum of options. In the notional case depicted in the figure, the rescue model first compares the results of combining fixed DCS teams and both types of aircraft nodes at an N+1 alert time at all locations (A through Z). Of all asset-location pairings compared in the first notional model run, the rotary-wing aircraft node at Location D offers the highest marginal benefit: a 0.91-percent increase in the expected survival rate (highlighted in the left table of the figure).

Figure 5.3
Spectrum of Asset-Location Pairings Considered

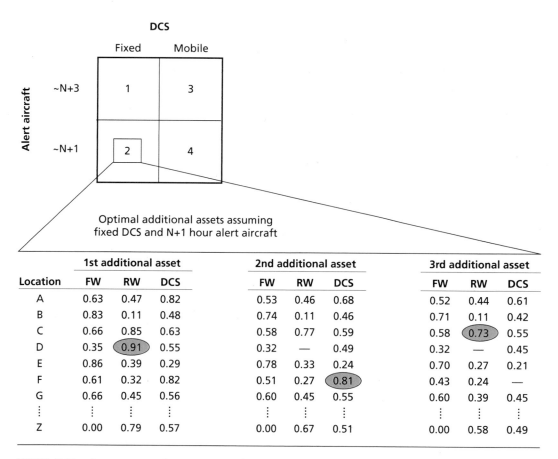

Location	1st additional asset			2nd additional asset			3rd additional asset		
	FW	RW	DCS	FW	RW	DCS	FW	RW	DCS
A	0.63	0.47	0.82	0.53	0.46	0.68	0.52	0.44	0.61
B	0.83	0.11	0.48	0.74	0.11	0.46	0.71	0.11	0.42
C	0.66	0.85	0.63	0.58	0.77	0.59	0.58	0.73	0.55
D	0.35	0.91	0.55	0.32	—	0.49	0.32	—	0.45
E	0.86	0.39	0.29	0.78	0.33	0.24	0.70	0.27	0.21
F	0.61	0.32	0.82	0.51	0.27	0.81	0.43	0.24	—
G	0.66	0.45	0.56	0.60	0.45	0.55	0.60	0.39	0.45
⋮	⋮	⋮	⋮	⋮	⋮	⋮	⋮	⋮	⋮
Z	0.00	0.79	0.57	0.00	0.67	0.51	0.00	0.58	0.49

NOTES: DCS = damage control surgery; FW = fixed-wing; RW = rotary-wing.
RAND RR2161z1-5.3

small marginal amount of this additional cost relative to the underlying cost uncertainty of a factor of two that we found for all assets being compared, the cost of decreased alert times is not explicitly included in our cost analysis.

Once this first optimal additional asset is placed at its respective location, the rescue model seeks the next optimal additional asset, which turns out to be a fixed DCS team at Location F (highlighted in the middle table of the figure), offering an additional 0.81-percent increase in the expected survival rate. Once these first two optimal additional assets are placed at their respective locations, the rescue model identifies the third optimal additional asset. In this hypothetical example, the third optimal additional asset is a rotary-wing aircraft node at Location C (highlighted in the right table of the figure), offering an additional 0.73-percent increase in the expected survival rate. The rescue model continues to identify the rest of the optimal marginal assets under these conditions (fixed DCS teams and N+1 alert times). Once the cycle is complete, the model can perform similar calculations for the remaining sets of conditions illustrated in the figures two-by-two quadrant, such as mobile DCS teams and N+3 alert times, and so on. The next section will shift the focus from notional to actual marginal increases in expected survival rates.

Marginal Increases in Expected Survival Rates

The next four charts walk through the most cost-effective marginal investments under different sets of conditions and choices, showing each incremental increase in the expected survival rate from each optimal choice. For instance, Figure 5.4 represents each optimal choice from among three alternatives: fixed-wing aircraft on standard alert times, rotary-wing aircraft on standard alert times, or fixed DCS teams.[4] The figure shows the first eight results from adding each remaining alternative to the locations and comparing the cost-effectiveness scores across the asset-location pairings. The model recalculates the comparative scores all over again for each marginal increment, factoring in the previously selected optimal investments. In all cases, the model sets the standard alert times at N+3 for additional fixed-wing or rotary-wing aircraft. Given the three choices, according to the model, the first most cost-effective additional asset-location pairing would be a new DCS team. With the new DCS team incorporated into the model, it then calculates the next optimal marginal investment, which would be another DCS team. With both of those DCS teams incorporated into the model, it calculates the subsequent optimal marginal investment, and so on. In this case, under these assumptions of standard alert times and fixed DCS teams, all eight of the optimal marginal capabilities would be DCS teams, as opposed to aircraft, dispersed across the operational area. This striking result could call into question the value of the standard alert times for rescue missions. Once the DCS team is established, the model

---

[4]   We explored the sensitivity of these results to whether or not the population in Djibouti was included. When excluding the population in Djibouti, the range between the baseline and minimum risk postures is expanded, and the survival curve with increased capabilities is stretched out, but the findings remain qualitatively unchanged.

Figure 5.4
Optimal Additional Assets, Given Standard Alert Times and Fixed DCS

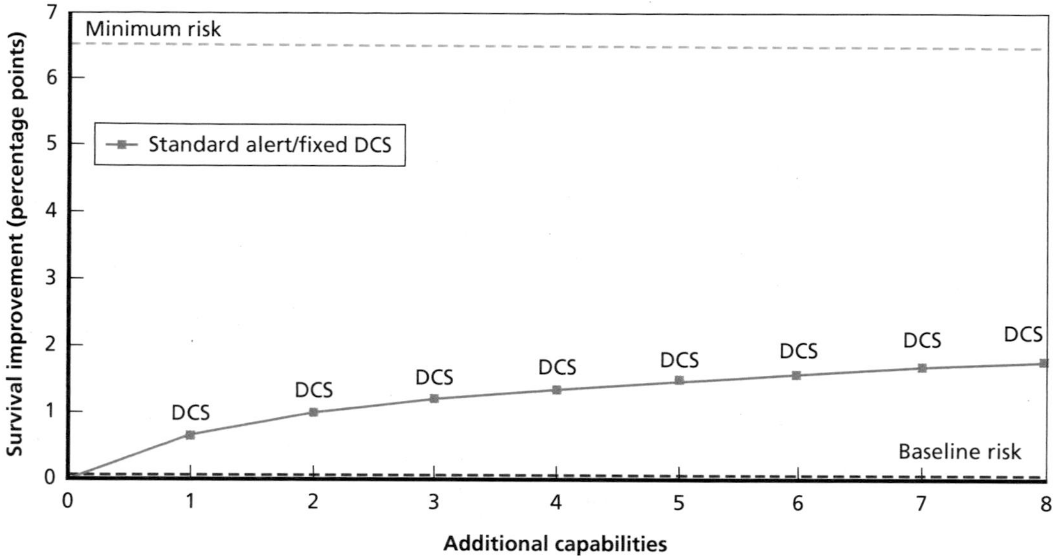

NOTE: DCS = damage control surgery.
RAND RR2161z1-5.4

suggests that each additional DCS team would offer a marginal improvement in the average estimated survival rate of about 0.1 percent.

We then alter one assumption: We shorten the aircraft alert times to N+1, which means, for most dedicated assets, the injured person reaches surgical care two hours faster. We still compare the cost-effectiveness of both kinds of aircraft with that of a fixed DCS capability at all locations. This change only modestly raises the estimated survival rates across the range of optimal additional capabilities, as seen in Figure 5.5. Relative to maintaining the standard aircraft alert times with fixed DCS teams, reducing the alert times to N+1 while relying on just the same fixed DCS teams results in all eight of the optimal additional investments still being fixed DCS teams. Decreasing the alert times alone yields about a 0.3-percent increase in the expected survival rates across the board (the height of the purple line above the orange line). Thus, the marginal cost-effectiveness of decreasing alert times alone is negligible, according to the model. The order of preference in the succession of additional DCS teams is also left largely unchanged.

Next, we alter just the other initial assumption: We replace the fixed DCS teams with mobile DCS teams. When a DCS team can move forward to a patient's location, the patient can receive surgical care faster and hence move up more quickly to a role 2 curve that offers higher survivability. The model compares the marginal effects of the mobile DCS team with those of additional aircraft on standard alert times. The results appear in Figure 5.6. Doing nothing but making the DCS capabilities mobile

Figure 5.5
Optimal Additional Assets, Given Shortened Alert Times and Fixed DCS

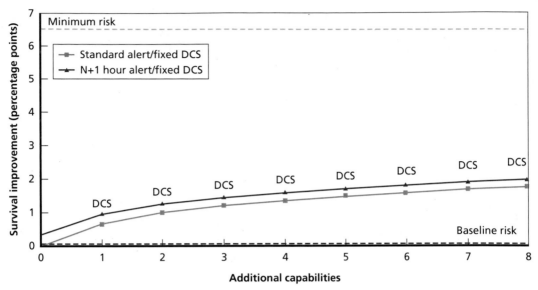

NOTE: DCS = damage control surgery.

RAND RR2161z1-5.5

at the U.S. MTF locations on the continent would spur a larger increase in the average expected survival rate than would decreasing the aircraft alert times to N+1. Again, though, the marginal benefits across the eight optimal additional asset-location pairings would be small. Relative to relying on fixed DCS teams, relying on mobile teams would raise the average expected survival rates about 0.7 percent across the board. There is one intriguing difference, however: With mobile DCS capabilities in place at the first six additional locations, the standard-alert aircraft now become the most cost-effective investments at the seventh and eighth locations. In addition, the availability of mobile DCS teams scrambles the order of optimal locations.

Finally, we alter both of the initial assumptions: We replace the standard alert times with N+1 alert times at all locations, and we replace the fixed DCS teams with mobile DCS teams at each location.[5] Combining the shorter alert times with the mobile DCS capability produces a bigger, nonlinear jump in expected survival rates. Whereas changing just the first assumption raises the expected survival rate by 0.3 percent and changing just the second assumption raises the expected survival rate by 0.7 percent relative to the baseline, changing both assumptions raises the expected survival rate by 2.2 percent relative to the baseline. As a result, even without a single additional

---

[5] The additional cost of alert times is not explicitly captured in this analysis. Discussions with a private contractor suggest that achieving N+1 hour or faster alert times for existing contracted PR nodes in AFRICOM would increase the cost of those nodes by about 20 percent.

Figure 5.6
Optimal Additional Assets, Given Standard Alert Times and Mobile DCS

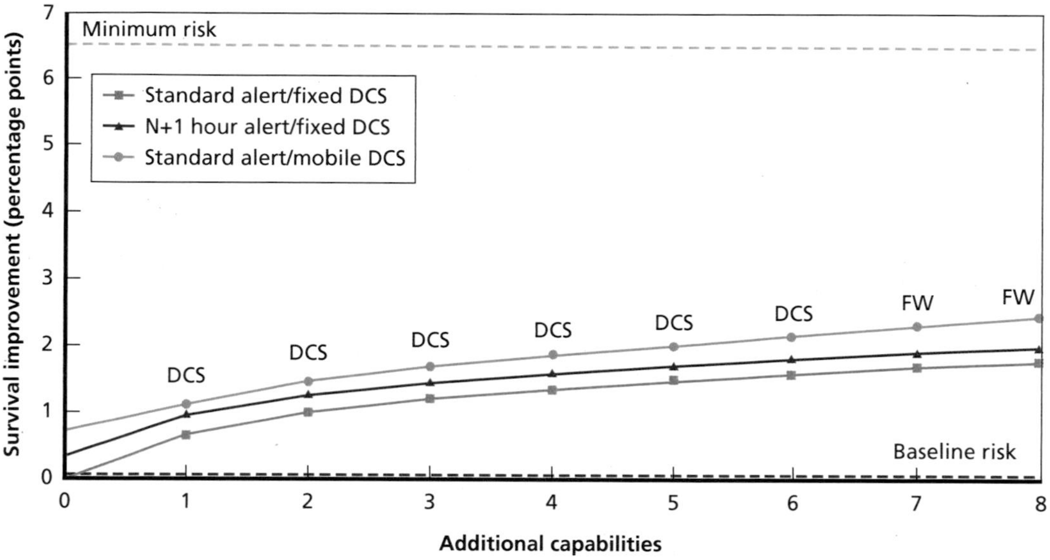

NOTES: DCS = damage control surgery; FW = fixed-wing.
RAND RR2161z1-5.6

asset, mobile DCS teams combined with shortened alert times produce an equal or better outcome than all eight optimal additional investments under the other sets of conditions. Once again, with mobile DCS teams in place, the fixed-wing and rotary-wing aircraft nodes assume greatest marginal importance for subsequent investments. Figure 5.7 shows the results.

Figure 5.8 makes the nonlinearity of the gains from mobile DCS teams more obvious. Recall that the minimum risk case is defined as a DCS facility, an N+1 helicopter, and an N+6 C-17 plane at more than 500 airfields across the AFRICOM AOR. The four points on the vertical axis in Figure 5.7 correspond with four points along the curves in Figure 5.8, specifically both points in Figure 5.8 set at three hours and both set at one hour. Figure 5.8 makes clear that if DCS capabilities are fixed, then there is little benefit to be gained from decreasing aircraft alert times. However, if DCS capabilities are mobile, there is an exponential benefit to be gained from decreasing aircraft alert times, especially with those shorter than an hour. If mobile DCS teams could somehow be combined with rescue aircraft placed on alert times of N+0, then about three-quarters of the rescue posture gap could be filled.

It would certainly be a challenge to cut the alert times of rescue aircraft to N+5 minutes. Nonetheless, these findings suggest the potential for harnessing the nonlinear gains promised by shorter aircraft alert times when combined with mobile DCS teams. These findings could be applied to other model runs involving other types of aircraft, other types of locations, and other underlying assumptions.

Figure 5.7
Optimal Additional Assets, Given Shortened Alert Times and Mobile DCS

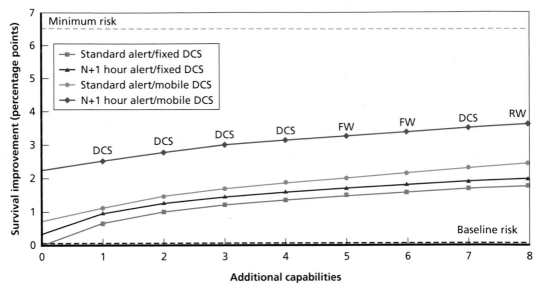

NOTES: DCS = damage control surgery; FW = fixed-wing; RW = rotary-wing.
RAND RR2161z1-5.7

Figure 5.8
Importance of Shortened Aircraft Alert Times

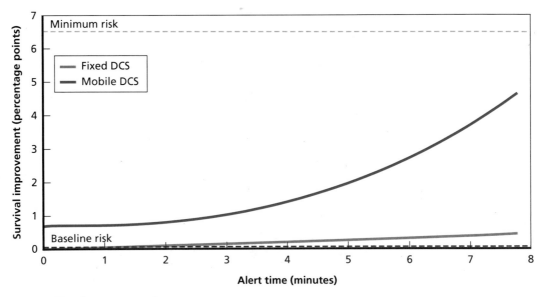

NOTE: DCS = damage control surgery.
RAND RR2161z1-5.8

Key Findings from the Cost-Effectiveness Comparisons

Three key findings emerge from the foregoing comparison of investment options:

1. There is a very strong synergy to be gained from combining mobile DCS teams with shorter aircraft alert times (e.g., N+1).
2. These synergies increase rapidly with decreasing alert times below one hour. Compared with a notional alert time of three hours, an alert time of 15 minutes would be more than twice as beneficial as an alert time of one hour. The expected survival rate would rise 1.5 percentage points going from three hours' notice to one hour's notice and 3.4 percentage points going from three hours' notice to 15 minutes' notice.
3. Additional DCS teams are always initially preferred to additional aircraft.

A fourth finding pertains to host-nation hospitals. Beyond their unsuitability for force planning purposes because of the risk of transmitting infectious diseases, host-nation hospitals would fare poorly, in terms of raising expected survival rates, even in comparison with fixed DCS teams and standard aircraft alert times. The reason why host-nation hospitals offer little potential benefit for raising expected survival rates, according to the rescue model, is that they are geographically separated from most of the PAR. Figure 5.9 shows the results for host-nation hospitals compared with those for the fixed DCS teams and standard alert times from Figure 5.4.[6]

---

[6] Although the benefit of partner nations' hospitals would appear to be small, if the cost associated with ensuring that they met quality-of-care standards were also small, or if they could provide care beyond that of a role 2 MTF, they could prove to be cost-effective options.

Figure 5.9
Host-National Hospitals Versus Fixed DCS Teams, Standard Alert Times

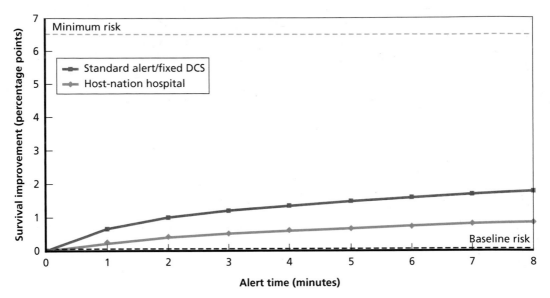

NOTE: DCS = damage control surgery.

RAND RR2161z1-5.9

CHAPTER SIX

Recommendations

The foregoing analysis points toward three recommendations for AFRICOM regarding cost-effective options for improving rescue, as follows:

1. Coordinate with DCS providers (Air Combat Command, Air Force Special Operations Command, Air Mobility Command, Army Medical Department, Navy Bureau of Medicine, and others) to ensure that mobile DCS teams can move surgical capabilities to patients during rescue missions.
2. Decrease the alert times of dedicated rescue aircraft to one hour.
3. Explore the feasibility of decreasing the alert times to less than one hour. The times can vary by location and can be adjusted, based on the estimated risk to force. The rescue aircraft and DCS teams can also be forward-staged to support high-risk activities in high-intensity zones of operation. These are just some of the options that can be explored.

Beyond these particular recommendations, future research could look at potential ways to radically expand the band of potential survival illustrated in Figure 5.2. Although beyond the scope of this research, such options may provide benefits that exceed the few percentage-point gains promised by the recommendations above. These options could include the following:

1. A role 3 ("theater hospital") facility on the African continent, potentially with the ability for the facility itself to be mobile—i.e., move to the patient's location. There is also the potential that such a capability could be assigned to a dedicated aircraft, allowing for the onboard medical capabilities necessary to provide role 3 care in the field.
2. The provision of more rapid, but less-than-surgical, levels of care. This capability could be similar to the Marine Corps' shock trauma platoons, for example, but with the added ability to be mobile and to move to the patient's location.
3. The enhancement of initial medical care delivered to injured personnel in the field.

Future work could also account for personnel whose presence in Africa might not be reflected in this analysis because of data limitations we encountered. With broader personnel data, it might also be possible for the rescue model to differentiate among the very different levels of personnel risk being experienced simultaneously by those serving at different operating locations across Africa and performing different operational activities from those locations.

References

Alion Science & Technology, Inc., subcontract 1137617 to Erickson Helicopters, Inc., November 4, 2014.

Bureau of Labor Statistics, website, undated. As of August 29, 2018:
http://www.bls.gov

Carlton, Maj Gen P. K., and Maj John Pilcher, "The Mobile Field Surgical Team (MFST): A Surgical Team for Combat Casualty Care in the Information Age," paper presented at the AGARD AMP Symposium on "Aeromedical Support Issues in Contingency Operations," Rotterdam, the Netherlands, September 29–October 1, 1997.

Cusumano, Eugenio, "Money for Nothing? Contractor Support from an Economic Perspective," in Joakim Berndtsson and Christopher Kinsey, eds., *The Routledge Research Companion to Security Outsourcing*, New York: Routledge, 2016, pp. 76–85.

Defense Travel Management Office, website, undated. As of September 26, 2018:
http://www.defensetravel.dod.mil

Department of Defense Directive 3002.01, *Personnel Recovery in the Department of Defense*, Washington, D.C.: U.S. Department of Defense, May 24, 2017.

Ervin, Mark D., "Air Force Special Operations Command Special Operations Surgical Team (SOST) CONOPS," *Journal of Special Operations Medicine*, Vol. 8, No. 2, Spring 2008.

International SOS—*See* International SOS Government Services, Inc.

International SOS Government Services, Inc., "Government Services Business Expands with New TRICARE Program," September 23, 2015. As of August 29, 2018:
http://www.internationalsos.com/newsroom/news-releases/
government-services-business-expands-with-new-tricare-program-sep-23-2015

———, "Founders," 2017. As of August 29, 2018:
http://www.internationalsos.com/about-us/philosophy-and-values/founders

Irish, John, and Daniel Flynn, "France Seeks to Shed Its Policeman Role in Africa Meeting," Reuters, December 4, 2013.

Jayaraman, Sudha, Zaid Chalabi, Pablo Perel, C. Guerriero, and Ian Roberts, "The Risk of Transfusion-Transmitted Infection in Sub-Saharan Africa," *Transfusion Complications*, Vol. 50, February 2010, pp. 433–442.

JMPT—*See* Teledyne Brown Engineering, Inc., *Joint Medical Planning Tool Methodology Manual*, Huntsville, Ala., Version 8.1, 2015.

Joint Commission, "Facts About Joint Commission International," July 20, 2016. As of August 29, 2018:
http://www.jointcommission.org/facts_about_joint_commission_international/

Joint Commission International, *Accreditation Standards for Hospitals, Including Standards for Academic Medical Center Hospitals*, 5th Edition, Oak Brook, Ill.: Joint Commission International, April 1, 2014.

Joint Publication 3-50, *Personnel Recovery*, Washington, D.C.: Joint Chiefs of Staff, October 23, 2017.

Joint Publication 4-02, *Health Service Support*, Washington, D.C.: Joint Chiefs of Staff, July 26, 2012.

Lurie, Philip M., *Comparing the Costs of Military Treatment Facilities with Private Sector Care*, Alexandria, Va.: Institute for Defense Analyses, February 2016.

Martin, Guy, "AAR Awarded U.S. Military African Airlift Contract," defenceWeb, December 4, 2013.

McCann, John, "Graphic: US Military's Presence in Africa," *Mail & Guardian*, September 17, 2018.

Mitchell, Ray, Mike Galarneau, Bill Hancock, and Doug Lowe, *Modeling Dynamic Casualty Mortality Curves in the Tactical Medical Logistics (TML+) Planning Tool*, San Diego, Calif.: Naval Health Research Center, October 2004.

Mouton, Christopher, and John P. Godges, *Timelines for Reaching Injured Personnel in Africa*, Santa Monica, Calif.: RAND Corporation, RR-1536-OSD, 2016. As of August 14, 2018: https://www.rand.org/pubs/research_reports/RR1536.html

Mouton, Christopher A., John P. Godges, and Edward W. Chan, *Improving Rescue Capabilities in the AFRICOM AOR: The Need for a New Approach*, Santa Monica, Calif.: RAND Corporation, 2018, not available to the general public.

National Center for Medical Intelligence, homepage, undated. As of August 29, 2018: http://www.ncmi.detrick.army.mil/aboutafmic.php

———, Blood Safety Index, 2017.

Naval Health Research Center, Document Number 09-6F, *Air Force Operational Medicine, Using the Estimating Supplies Program to Develop Materiel Solutions for the Operational Clinical Requirements of the Expeditionary Medical Support (EMEDS) System*, Volume One: *The Small Portable Expeditionary Aeromedical Rapid Response (SPEARR) System*, undated.

Naval Health Research Center, *Medical Planners' Toolkit (MPTk)*, San Diego, Calif., 2013.

Naval Health Research Center and Teledyne Brown Engineering, Inc., *Medical Planners' Toolkit*, Version 1.2.0.17, developed for the Defense Health Agency, 2016.

NCMI—*See* National Center for Medical Intelligence.

Preston, Samuel H., and Emily Buzzell, "Mortality of American Troops in Iraq," University of Pennsylvania, PSC Working Paper Series, August 26, 2006.

Salary.com, website, undated. As of August 29, 2018: http://www.salary.com

Technical Manual TM 8-227-12, *Armed Services Blood Program, Joint Blood Program Handbook*, Washington, D.C.: Departments of the Army, the Navy, and the Air Force, December 1, 2011.

Teledyne Brown Engineering, Inc., *Joint Medical Planning Tool Methodology Manual*, Huntsville, Ala., Version 8.1, 2015.

Trauma Society of South Africa, "Trauma Care Accreditation," 2017. As of August 29, 2018: http://www.traumasa.co.za/trauma-centre-accreditation/

TRICARE, "TRICARE Overseas Program Prime Remote," fact sheet, August 2016.

U.S. Department of Defense, *Department of Defense Dictionary of Military and Associated Terms*, November 8, 2010 (amended February 15, 2016).

U.S. Department of State, website, undated. As of August 29, 2018:
http://www.state.gov

U.S. Department of State, Bureau of Consular Affairs, "Doctors/Hospitals Abroad," undated. As of August 29, 2018:
https://web.archive.org/web/20170101002433/travel.state.gov/content/passports/en/go/health/doctors.html

U.S. Navy contract N00189-14-C-0056 to AAR Airlift Group, Inc., June 10, 2014.

U.S. Special Operations Command Request for Information H92222-16-R-NSRW, March 2016.

U.S. Transportation Command contract HTC711-13-D-C013 to Berry Aviation, Inc., July 25, 2013.

World Health Organization, "Launch of WHO Collaborative Centre on Patient Safety Solutions," August 2005. As of August 29, 2018:
https://web.archive.org/web/20170717071444/http://www.who.int/patientsafety/newsalert/issue2/en/